DIET AND ATHEROSCLEROSIS

ADVANCES IN EXPERIMENTAL MEDICINE AND BIOLOGY

Recent Volumes in this Series

Volume 50
ION-SELECTIVE MICROELECTRODES
Edited by Herbert J. Berman and Normand C. Hebert • 1974

Volume 51
THE CELL SURFACE: Immunological and Chemical Approaches
Edited by Barry D. Kahan and Ralph A. Reisfeld • 1974

Volume 52
HEPARIN: Structure, Function, and Clinical Implications
Edited by Ralph A. Bradshaw and Stanford Wessler • 1975

Volume 53
CELL IMPAIRMENT IN AGING AND DEVELOPMENT
Edited by Vincent J. Cristofalo and Emma Holečková • 1975

Volume 54
BIOLOGICAL RHYTHMS AND ENDOCRINE FUNCTION
Edited by Laurence W. Hedlund, John M. Franz, and
Alexander D. Kenny • 1975

Volume 55
CONCANAVALIN A
Edited by Tushar K. Chowdhury and A. Kurt Weiss • 1975

Volume 56
BIOCHEMICAL PHARMACOLOGY OF ETHANOL
Edited by Edward Majchrowicz • 1975

Volume 57
THE SMOOTH MUSCLE OF THE ARTERY
Edited by Stewart Wolf and Nicholas T. Werthessen • 1975

Volume 58
CYTOCHROMES P-450 and b_5: Structure, Function, and Interaction
Edited by David Y. Cooper, Otto Rosenthal, Robert Snyder,
and Charlotte Witmer • 1975

Volume 59
ALCOHOL INTOXICATION AND WITHDRAWAL: Experimental Studies II
Edited by Milton M. Gross • 1975

Volume 60
DIET AND ATHEROSCLEROSIS
Edited by Cesare Sirtori, Giorgio Ricci, and Sergio Gorini • 1975

DIET AND ATHEROSCLEROSIS

Edited by

Cesare Sirtori

Institute of Pharmacology
University of Milan
Milan, Italy

Giorgio Ricci

Institute for Systematic Medical Therapy
University of Rome
Rome, Italy

and

Sergio Gorini

Giovanni Lorenzini Foundation
Milan, Italy

PLENUM PRESS • NEW YORK AND LONDON

Library of Congress Cataloging in Publication Data

International Course on Diet and Atherosclerosis, Rome, 1973.
    Diet and atherosclerosis.

    (Advances in experimental medicine and biology; v. 60)
    Includes bibliographical references and index.
    1. Arteriosclerosis—Congresses. 2. Diet in disease—Congresses. I. Sirtori, Cesare.
II. Ricci, Giorgio. III. Gorini, S. IV. Title. V. Series. [DNLM: 1. Diet,
Atherogenic—Congresses. 2. Arteriosclerosis—Congresses. W1 AD559 v. 60/
WG550 D565 1973]
RC692.I47 1973   616.1'36'071   75-15608
ISBN 0-306-39060-4

Proceedings of the International Course on Diet and Atherosclerosis,
held in Rome, Italy, November 1-3, 1973

© 1975 Plenum Press, New York
A Division of Plenum Publishing Corporation
227 West 17th Street, New York, N.Y. 10011

United Kingdom edition published by Plenum Press, London
A Division of Plenum Publishing Company, Ltd.
Davis House (4th floor), 8 Scrubs Lane, Harlesden, London, NW10 6SE, England

Printed in the United States of America

FOREWORD

The papers in the present volume were presented on November
1st-3rd, 1973, in Rome on the occasion of an International Post-
graduate Course sponsored by the Italian Society for the Study of
Atherosclerosis, the Istituto Superiore di Sanità, and the
Fondazione Giovanni Lorenzini.

The purpose of this course was to gather information and to
draw attention to the role of diet in the pathogenesis of experimental and human arteriosclerosis, as well as its prevention and
therapy.

Konrad Bloch, in the opening lecture, emphasized the features
unique to fatty acid synthesis in animal tissues and discussed the
importance of comparative biochemical research in the study of
control mechanisms of lipid biosynthesis.

The lectures in the morning were followed in the afternoon by
short practical demonstrations (R. Angelico, O. Lostia, A. Menotti,
D.H. Blankenhorn, A. Ferro Luzzi).

Particular attention was paid to the problem of dietary edu-
cation in Italy, during a round-table discussion on November 2nd
(G. Bergami, G. Ricci, G. Crepaldi, F. Fidanza, S.F. Feruglio,
M. Proia, A. Mariani, L. Ribolzi).

The educational purpose of the course is obvious in Italy, a
country where the people had been accustomed for centuries to the
intake of a virtually nonatherogenic diet, until, quite recently,
the migration from agricultural to industrialized areas assumed
sociologically significant levels. It was then found that the
lipoproteinemic patterns of the migrated population had shifted
toward higher levels.

Experimentally, it is possible to induce atherosclerosis in
rabbits and in baboons by feeding them semisynthetic diets rich
in carbohydrates and saturated fats and free of cholesterol (the
addition of saturated fats to laboratory chow does not render the

chow atherogenic); the resulting hypercholesterolemia may be the
result of the reduced synthesis of biliary acids (D. Kritchevsky).
Serum triglyceride concentration is increased, together with prebetalipoproteins in spontaneously diabetic monkeys (C.F. Howard
Jr.). Serum triglycerides are sensitive to the amount and type of
carbohydrates in the diet. The type of fat bound to carbohydrates
may modify the response of triglyceride levels (I. MacDonald).

The atherogenic effect of saturated fats may be increased by
adding some vegetable oils (coconut oil, peanut oil) to the diet
of monkeys, which also influences the morphology of the arterial
lesions (R.W. Wissler). Morphological effects on the arterial wall
may be elicited ("edematous reaction" through contraction and
phagocyting activity of endothelial cells) by drugs and diet
(T. Shimamoto).

Platelets and blood coagulation are also influenced by lipids
and fatty acids. Saturated fatty acids are activators of the "contact factor" in the intrinsic clotting system and exert an influence on the activation of platelets, as do prostaglandins (E.F.
Lüscher). Phospholipids of red blood cells and phospholipids and
fatty acids of platelets may differ in nutritionally different
areas (Cincinnati, Ohio; Milan and Palermo, Italy) and the lipid
composition of platelets may have an effect on their function; the
nutritional state may predispose to thrombogenic phenomena
(J.M. Iacono et al.).

Diet-related risk factors were discussed by J. Stamler, while
J.C. Somogyi, R. Angelico, and M. Mancini presented lectures concerning the prevention and therapy of atherosclerosis by diet.
Whatever the opinions, restriction of dietary cholesterol is extremely important in preventing atherosclerosis, as underlined by
P.H. Schreibman, as well as in promoting the reversal of advanced
atherosclerotic lesions, as stated by R.W. Wissler. In rhesus
monkeys passing from a severely atherogenic diet to a diet devoid
of cholesterol and containing small amounts of polyunsaturated fats
the arterial lesions regressed consistently.

In birds, reversion of experimental atherosclerosis was bene-
ficially influenced by physical exercise, as noted by Y. C. Wong.

The diagnostic methods proposed by D.H. Blankenhorn to ascertain safely the degree of arterial lesions in living subjects
may therefore be very important not only in diagnosing the degree
of parietal lesion, but also in determing the degree of lesion
reversal.

> Giorgio Weber
> President
> Italian Society for the
> Study of Atherosclerosis

PREFACE

After the success of the two previous meetings on Typing of
Hyperlipoproteinemias, in Milan in 1971 and in Rome in 1972, an
important part of each of which was devoted to the discussion of
therapy, the Italian Society for the Study of Atherosclerosis,
the Istituto Superiore di Sanità, and the Fondazione Giovanni
Lorenzini planned a special treatment of this important topic.
This meeting was held in Rome in November 1973 at the Istituto
Superiore di Sanità. On this occasion the most important subjects developed in recent years by the most qualified centers
of experimental and clinical research were reported.

A broad discussion took place regarding the role of diet in
causing or worsening the biohumoral changes and the lesions peculiar to arteriosclerosis, while other distinguished authors reported on the role of diet in delaying or correcting the dyslip-
idemic state.

We are deeply indebted to all the authors, whose superior
competence and unstinting effort made this course possible. We
express our thanks also to Plenum Press, since the printing of
these proceedings affords an important aid to those anxious and
willing to deepen their knowledge of this important subject.

Cesare Sirtori Jr.

Giorgio Ricci

Sergio Gorini

CONTENTS

Some Aspects of the Control of Lipid Biosynthesis . . .   1
   Konrad Bloch

The Relationship of Diet and Atherosclerosis in
       Diabetic <u>Macaca</u> <u>nigra</u>   13
   Charles F. Howard Jr.

The Effects of Physical Exercise in Reversing
       Experimental Atherosclerosis   33
   H.Y.C. Wong, S.N. David, S.O. Orimilikwe,
   and F.B. Johnson

Diet and Human Atherosclerosis - Carbohydrates   57
   I. MacDonald

The Effects of Feeding Various Dietary Fats on the
       Development and Regression of Hypercholes-
       terolemia and Atherosclerosis   65
   R.W. Wissler and D. Vesselinovitch

Drugs and Foods on Contraction of Endothelial Cells as
       a Key Mechanism in Atherogenesis and Treatment
       of Atherosclerosis with Endothelial-Cell
       Relaxants (Cyclic AMP Phosphodiesterase
       Inhibitors)   77
   T. Shimamoto

The Effects of Lipids and Fatty Acids on Blood
       Coagulation and Platelets in Relation to
       Thrombosis   107
   E. F. Lüscher

Diagnostic Methods for the Study of Human
       Atherosclerosis   119
   D. H. Blankenhorn

Diet-Related Risk Factors for Human Atherosclerosis:
        Hyperlipidemia, Hypertension, Hyper-
        glycemia -- Current Status   125
    J. Stamler

Diet and Plasma Lipids   159
    P. H. Schreibman

Outlines of Dietary Prevention of Atherosclerosis . . .   171
    R. Angelico

The Influence of Dietary Fats on Hypercoagulation
        and Thrombosis   191
    James M. Iacono

Prevention of Atherosclerosis by Diet: Present State
        and Conclusions   205
    J. C. Somogyi

The Effects of Feeding Various Carbohydrates on the
        Development of Hypercholesterolemia and
        Atherosclerosis   231
    David Kritchevsky

Index   251

SOME ASPECTS OF THE CONTROL OF LIPID BIOSYNTHESIS

KONRAD BLOCH

From the James Bryant Conant Laboratories
Harvard University
Cambridge, Massachusetts 02138 U.S.A.

It seems indisputable that the control and management of athe-rosclerosis, whether by diet or by chemotherapy will ultimately be founded on the scientific understanding of the metabolic aberrations that provoke the disease. Such a belief is perhaps difficult to sustain in view of the very slow and limited progress that has been made towards that goal over recent decades. Yet no alternatives or shortcuts present themselves. Our approaches cannot be guided by expediency. We cannot abandon the rigorous scientific principles which have been the basis of scholarship during modern times.

In reviewing Control Mechanisms of Lipid Metabolism, I fully acknowledge the possibility, however slight, that lipid-related metabolic defects or derangements in atherosclerosis may be second-ary consequences rather than primary causes of the disease. Be that as it may, the existence of this degenerative disease which threatens to assume epidemic proportions has provided a powerful stimulus for research in the lipid field.

The successful charting of metabolic maps during the last four decades, primarily with the aid of the isotopic tracer technique, microbial mutants and the highly developed art of enzymology has also led to a very detailed knowledge of lipid chemistry and meta-bolism. We can, of course, never be certain that the catalogue of known compounds and pathways is complete and must anticipate the future discovery of novel lipids, either variants of established classes or molecules of an entirely new type. As examples I need only mention the prostaglandins, the polyisoprenoid hydrocarbon dolichol or the more complex glycolipids.

Turning first to the control of cholesterol biosynthesis, I need not remind you of the intricacies of this process except to point out that the unravelling of the sequential steps in the transformation of acetyl-CoA to mevalonic acid was an essential prelude to the recognition of one of the important control points in cholesterol biogenesis. In retrospect, it is equally clear that without the concept of negative feedback control in the background, Gould's observations in 1953 on cholesterol inhibition of cholesterol biosynthesis (7) would have been baffling and paradoxical. Impressive evidence has since accumulated that beta-hydroxy-beta-methylglutaryl-CoA (HMG-CoA) reductase catalyzes the rate-controlling step in cholesterol biosynthesis and that the synthesis of this enzyme is subject to end product inhibition (17). Changes in overall rate, whether due to cholesterol feeding, starvation, diabetes or Triton injection all seem to correlate well with fluctuating levels of the hepatic microsomal HMG-CoA reductase. Unfortunately, the detailed mechanism of this inhibition has so far eluded analysis because the phenomenon is demonstrable only in vivo. It involves the largely obscure processes of enzyme synthesis, i.e., induction and repression rather than allosteric regulation of enzyme activity.

One of the most intriguing aspects of HMG-CoA reductase regulation is the circadian fluctuation of this activity which Kandutsch discovered in 1969 (8). Both the hypophysis and the adrenal gland seem to provide the hormonal signals for synthesis of the enzyme but neither the identity of the hormones involved nor their mode of action have been uncovered (5). One should perhaps be mindful of the fact that this circadian rhythm has been studied and established only in certain experimental animals and it is not at all clear whether and how it is related to feeding schedules and other unrecognized environmental factors.

Control of HMG-CoA reductase, the rate-limiting enzyme, by the endproduct, cholesterol is a typical example of negative feed-back control. The enzyme produces mevalonate the first specific intermediate in the pathway by catalyzing what in current parlance is the "committed step". However attractive, this concept may be too simple because it neglects the fact that mevalonate is not only the precursor of cholesterol but also of several non-steroidal products. These quantitatively minor but physiologically important products include the polyisoprenol side chains of ubiquinone and dolichol, the lipid carrier in glycoprotein synthesis. Moreover, some recent evidence strongly suggests a branching of the main pathway at a stage prior to squalene leading to the estrogen-related equilin and equilenine directly rather than by way of cholesterol (1).

Mechanisms operating in the control of branched pathways have been studied extensively in bacterial amino acid biosynthesis. For dealing with such complex regulatory situations, nature appears to have invented two principal devices. One is multivalent repression or inhibition of the enzyme catalyzing the committed step. Each of the several end products of the branched pathway inhibits the enzyme or its synthesis partially but the effects are additive. Alternatively, the enzyme catalyzing the committed step may exist in multiple forms, each susceptible to one end product of the branched pathway but not to others. It, therefore, seems entirely possible that the microsomal HMG-CoA reductase is either subject to multiple end product inhibition or that it exists in several independent forms. Since we are dealing with the control of HMG-CoA reductase synthesis rather than allosteric regulation of enzyme activity, no easy solution of this problem is in sight.

Very recently interest has focused on still earlier control sites in the sterol pathway. According to the important findings of Lane et. al. (3), beta-ketoacyl thiolase and HMG-CoA synthetase occur in the cytoplasm as well as in the mitochondria. A cytoplasmic provision of acetoacetyl-CoA and HMG-CoA would first of all make sterol synthesis autonomous and independent of the mitochondrial supply of these precursors. At the same time HMG-CoA would lose its status as the common intermediate in both ketogenesis and cholesterol synthesis. It seems significant in this context that the citric acid analogue, hydroxycitrate, not only blocks hepatic cholesterogenesis but also inhibits ATP: citrate lyase, the enzyme that supplies extramitochondrial acetyl-CoA. The cytoplasmic thiolase-synthetase system, therefore, emerges as a major and possibly specific source of precursors for HMG-CoA. Cholesterol feeding also represses the synthesis of these two cytoplasmic enzymes, the synthetase more so than the thiolase. While these enzymes are less sensitive to cholesterol repression than HMG-CoA reductase, they are at least potentially loci for an adaptive, secondary mechanism of regulation. These findings are too recent to allow any assessment or reassessment of the main control sites in cholesterol biosynthesis. What one would wish to know inter alia is whether cytoplasmic thiolase and HMG-CoA synthetase show a similar circadian pattern as HMG-CoA reductase and whether they respond in a like manner to the various changes in physiological state.

Next, I would like to raise the question whether any control mechanisms operate past the mevalonate stage. I am unaware of any experimental evidence to date for a physiologically significant regulation of the intermediate steps between mevalonic acid and cholesterol, either by repression, induction or allosterically. In the early stages the intracellular locale of cholesterol biosynthesis shifts back and forth between the cytoplasm and the endoplasmic reticulum but from farnesylpyrophosphate on all steps are

catalyzed by microsomal enzymes, several of them of the mixed-
function oxygenase type. Some of the latter, most likely components of the demethylase system, contain cytochrome P-450 as the
prosthetic group. It is, therefore, somewhat unexpected that the
p-450 oxygenases of the sterol pathway appear not to be inducible
by barbiturates or carcinogenic hydrocarbons. They do not share
this interesting property with the various drug metabolizing enzymes of the mixed oxygenase type.

    A recently discovered and still somewhat controversial pheno-
menon is the participation of certain non-catalytic proteins in
one or more steps between squalene and cholesterol (15, 16, 20).
Two or possibly three such porteins appear to exist. They are referred to by some authors as Sterol-Carrier Proteins (SCP; 15, 16)
while we prefer a less specific terminology (soluble protein factor, SPF (20). Squalene epoxidase and 7-dehydro-cholesterol reductase are the only individual steps that have so far been shown
to respond to these proteins. Stimulations of microsomal enzyme
preparations in the range of 5-10 fold can be demonstrated. The
SCP preparation isolated by Ritter and Dempsey is replaceable by
human high density apo-lipoprotein but apparently not identical
with it (15). On the other hand, the SCP described by Scallen et.
al (16) is said to have properties similar to low-density lipoprotein (LDL). SCP is thought to fuction as substrate carrier,
promoting interactions of dispersed water-insoluble intermediates
with membrane-associated enzymes. Experiments describing the binding of various biosynthetic intermediates to SCP have been reported
(15,16) but unfortunately the binding specificity is relatively low.
On the other hand, the soluble protein isolated in our laboratory
that stimulates the microsomal expoxidation of squalene lacks any
binding ability for squalene or squalene-epoxide nor is it replaceable by Apo-HDL. We have further observed (14) that in the squa-
lene-epoxidase system the protein factor (SPF) can be replaced by
Triton X-100 and once the enzyme is solubilized, only the Triton
stimulation persists; the SPF effect disappears. The indications
that only microsomal or membrane-bound enzymes of the sterol pathway respond to SCP or SPF is indeed suggestive of a carrier function which, however, remains to be proven. There is little doubt
that these protein effects are real and reasonably specific but
their mode of action is far from clear nor are these non-catalytic
proteins necessarily significant for regulation. Nevertheless,
this aspect should be explored further and it should not be without interest to ascertain whether nutritional or hormonal conditions that affect rates of choesterol synthesis via induction or
repression also influence the levels of these auxiliary proteins.

    If one asks whether the investigation of cholesterol bio-
synthesis and metabolism and the resulting leads for the design

of potentially inhibitory substrate analogues have led to useful
applications for the management of atherosclerosis, the answer is
a definite no or, at least, not yet. Clofibrate and related hypolipidemic drugs are products of the time-honored and occasionally
successful empiricism of screening chemicals taken from the shelf.
Such agents could probably have been developed in the absence of any
basic understanding of cholesterol metabolism. The pharmaceutical
industry is certainly to be complimented for the design of effective hypolipidemic drugs. Yet one can not hide a sense of disap-
pointment over the failure of so-called basic research in provid-
ing the rationale for these successes.

My second topic has to do with the regulation of certain phases
of fatty acid biosynthesis. Here again, as in the case of cholesterol biosynthesis, the causal relation of biosynthetic rates to plasma levels of lipids and lipoproteins and in turn to arterial lipid
deposition is suggestive but far from proven. I, therefore, repeat
my disclaimer as to the relevance of these comments to the principal
topics of this Symposium.

The two familiar metabolic control mechanism, short term allosteric effects on enzyme activity and long-term adaptation by
modulation of enzyme protein synthesis, appear to operate also in
the synthesis of long-chain fatty acids. Before discussing specific sites where control is or might be exerted, I should like to
consider three distinguishable phases and classes of enzymes that
constitute what one might call the "lipogenic system". In the terminology I am proposing, Phase I enzymes furnish the building blocks
and electron donors for the chain-building process, acetyl-CoA,
malonyl-CoA and NADPH. These precursors are utilized and consumed
in Phase II, fatty acid synthesis proper. This is catalyzed by the
highly organized multienzyme complexes known as fatty acid synthetases. Lastly, we may designate as Phase III the terminal and cooperative processes of fatty acyl glyceride synthesis, among them
the fatty acyl CoA synthetases, fatty acyl transferases, etc. Control of lipogenesis may be exerted at one, two or all three of these stages and if there is multiple control some of the control processes may be coordinated. Too little is known about the regulation
of Phase III enzymes, the final assembly of phosphoglycerides and
triglycerides to warrant any discussion at this time. On the pro-
position that control occurs principally at the "committed" step
catalyzed by the first specific enzyme of the pathway we will wish
to focus attention on the components of Phase I, ATP-citrate lyase,
acetyl-CoA carboxylase or one or more of the NADPH generating enzymes.

The prime candidacy and strategic position of acetyl-CoA carboxylase in the control of fatty synthesis appears well established.
Firstly, the enzyme catalyzes the formation of malonyl-CoA, the intermediate that is used specifically for fatty acid synthesis but

not for any other pathway.   Secondly, the subunit structure and
other molecular properties of acetyl-CoA carboxylase are clearly
those of a regulatory enzyme.   Allosteric modifiers markedly influence its activity either positively (citrate and other Krebs
cycle intermediates) or negatively (palmitoyl-CoA) (23).   The se-
lection of citrate and palmitoyl-CoA as modifiers seems eminently
reasonably for the purposes of over-all metabolic regulation.
Citrate levels signal the degree of saturation of the Krebs cycle
and, therefore, of energy supply while palmitoyl-CoA, acting presumably as a negative feedback inhibitor, opposes the citrate effect by competing for the same enzyme site.   Nevertheless, there
is still some question whether acetyl-CoA carboxylase principally
or solely controls long-chain fatty acid synthesis.   This uncertain-
ty arises from quantitative considerations such as activator concentrations in the cytoplasm under various physiological conditions.
The K_m for citrate in acetyl-CoA carboxylase activation is 2-6 mM
whereas the estimated citrate concentration in the cytoplasm is 0.1
- 0.2 mM, at least one order of magnitude less.   If these values
truly reflect citrate levels at or near the site of acetyl-CoA carboxylase activity, they may be insufficient to activate carboxylase
fully in vivo.   Also, cytoplasmic citrate levels do not appear to
fluctuate sufficiently to account for the drastic changes in fatty
acid synthesis that occur in extreme nutritional states.   On the
other hand, the in vivo concentrations of palmitoyl-CoA, the negative carboxylase effector, are well within the range (15-150 µM)
in which the isolated enzyme is severely inhibited.   Still, there
is a tendency to regard inhibition by long-chain acyl-CoA as a non-
specific non-detergent effect and, indeed, palmitoyl-CoA adversely
effects many enzyme activities which are not obviously related to
lipogenesis.   Nevertheless, it would seem valid to argue that significant inhibition of a candidate enzyme by effector concentrations
in the physiological range cannot be dismissed as non-specific.   I
will return to this point later in the discussion of palmitoyl-CoA
effects on other enzyme systems.

        Investigations on the mode of action of plasma-lipid lowering
drugs also appear to support the role of acetyl-CoA carboxylase as
a control enzyme in lipogenesis.   Agents of the clofibrate type inhibit the enzyme in vitro, possibly by competing with citrate.   It
remains to be established whether the drugs when given in effective
hypolipidemic doses reach the tissue levels required for enzyme inhibition.

        Long-term or adaptive control plays an equal and perhaps even
more important role in regulating acetyl-CoA carboxylase.   There is
a highly positive correlation between carboxylase level and fatty
acid synthesis in response to changes in physiological state.   Enzyme levels are drastically lowered by starvation, diabetes and
high fat diets, and they are raised by carbohydrate, insulin and
in the obese state (10, 23).

Undoubtedly nutritional and hormonal effects on lipogenesis are closely related and interdependent but whether there exist specific lipogenic hormones and specifically whether insulin belongs into that category is not known or at least a matter of speculation. In the context of hormonal control, the role of the secondary messengers cyclic-AMP and cyclic-GMP in activating or deactivating lipogenic enzymes such as acetyl-CoA carboxylase is beginning to receive increasing attention.

The question to be raised next is whether alternative, additional or subsidiary control mechanism play a role in accelerating or diminishing lipogenesis. There has been growing evidence, to the point of certainty, that mitochondrial citric acid is the principal source of hepatic fatty acid carbon by way of the ATP-citrate lyase reaction (10). In a sense then fatty acid synthesis begins with the exit of mitochondrial citrate ot the cytoplasm. Presumably, citrate transport by itself is subject to some kind of control and, in fact, according to recent evidence, palmitoyl-CoA interferes with this process. Acting on citrate cytoplasmic ATP-citrate lyase then produces acetyl-CoA for the fatty acid synthetase in the same cellular compartment. Citrate cleavage activity or levels of this enzyme apparently fluctuate as widely in response to various nutritional states and hormonal signals as acetyl-CoA carboxylase (stimulation by carbohydrate feeding and insulin and depression by starvation, diabetes and high fat diets) and the response is in the same direction. These changes presumably are adaptive and reflect enzyme synthesis and degradation. Little appears to be known whether citrate lyase also responds to instantaneous allosteric modulation of the kind that effects acetyl-CoA carboxylase.

The pertinent literature conveys the impression that NADPH and the enzymes that produce it, malic enzyme, glucose-6-phosphate dehydrogenase and isocitric dehydrogenase rarely become rate-limiting in fatty acid synthesis. These dehydrogenases are frequently referred to as lipogenic enzymes, even though they supply NADPH for reductive biosynthesis generally rather than for fatty acid synthesis alone. One possible manifestation of a lipogenic role of a NADPH generating enzyme is the drastic decline of malic enzyme levels during starvation. This may contribute to the impairment of fatty acid synthesis under stringent conditions but the quantitative significance of this depletion is difficult to assess. As for allosteric regulation, most of the NADPH linked dehydrogenases show a marked sensitivity to inhibition by palmitoyl-CoA (21). While, as previously noted, the detergent-like properties of long-chain acyl-CoA derivatives complicate the interpretation of these effects, the possibility seems real that NADPH supply is in fact under negative feedback control by this type of molecule. Current experiments in our laboratory strongly support the specificity of palmitoyl-CoA inhibition in the case of glucose-6-phosphate dehydrogenase. In this instance the effects can be clearly differentiated from those of the detergent SDS.

The regulation of the fatty acid synthetase proper (Phase II of lipid synthesis) is under active investigation in my laboratory with enzyme systems from various microbes and unicellular plants. The results are of comparative interest but may have little bearing on the present discussion because the regulatory mechanisms for microbial fatty acid synthesis and for fatty acid synthesis in animal tissues appear to operate at quite different sites of control. Apart from the obvious absence of primary hormonal signals in bacteria, the following differences stand out. Only animal tissue acetyl-CoA carboxylase is activated by citric acid; bacterial, plant and yeast carboxylase do not respond to this type of allosteric modulation. Similarly, microbial acetyl-CoA carboxylases are much more resistant to inhibition by palmitoyl-CoA at least at the concentration which inhibit the hepatic enzyme. This lack in response to small effector molecules may well be related to the profound differences in molecular structure between the two types of carboxylases (23). Equally important for regulation, the animal fatty acid synthetases from whatever source (liver, adipose tissue, brain or mammary gland) produce free fatty acids rather than fatty acyl-CoA derivatives. Free fatty acids inhibit the animal fatty acid synthetases only very weakly if at all. This means that the synthetase itself does not produce a feedback inhibitor sensu strictu if, indeed, palmitoyl-CoA regulation of acetyl-CoA carboxylase and other lipogenic enzymes should prove to be physiologically significant.

The only known source of the CoA derivatives of long-chain fatty acids are the microsomal or mitochondrial long-chain acyl-CoA synthetases. These enzymes are essential for initiating a variety of biosynthetic processes which require activation of the fatty acyl carboxyl group. This is true for oleic acid synthesis, for the transacylation reactions in phospholipid and triglyceride formation for elongation of the fatty acyl chain and for the subsequent synthesis of polyunsaturated fatty acids. Judging from the elevated levels of the fatty acyl-CoA derivatives in starvation and diabetes it appears that the fatty acyl-CoA synthetase reaction is either poorly controlled or else that the various acyl-CoA utilizing reactions, including transport to the mitochondria for beta-oxidation, cannot keep pace with acyl-CoA production.

The possible role of palmitoyl-CoA thioesterase, an ubiquitous hydrolytic enzyme with a marked specificity for C_{16}- and C_{18}-CoA derivatives, in regulating long-chain acyl-CoA levels is another subject that has received far too little attention. The thioesterase is very active in liver cytoplasm and unless its levels should prove to be diminished in starvation and diabetes the accumulation of substantial amounts of palmitoyl-CoA in conditions of dietary or hormonal insufficiency are difficult to explain.

I have already mentioned that in microbial systems palmitoyl-CoA or related end products play a major role in regulating the fatty acid synthetase proper, presumably by negative feedback inhibition (9, 11).   For example, the synthetases from yeast (19) and Mycobacterium phlei (6) , display linear initial velocities only for very brief periods of time presumably because accumulating end-products block further progress of the reaction.   Linear reaction rates can, however, be maintained by various means including the addition of BSA (9, 11) , of certain mycobacterial polysaccharides (9), alpha- and beta-cyclodextrins and their alkyl derivatives (12), palmitoyl thioesterase (6) and phospholipid vesicles (19).   Our results suggest that the common mode of action of these reagents is to protect the fatty acid synthetase against inhibition or inactivation by palmitoyl-CoA.   This is achieved either by product hydrolysis (thioesterase), by removal of palmitoyl-CoA from the aqueous phase (phospholipid vesicles) or by tightly complexing palmitoyl-CoA in successful competition with the synthetase protein (BSA and polysaccharides).   There seems little doubt that palmitoyl-CoA is a generally important modifier of fatty acid synthesis.   However, the point which has emerged from the cited comparative studies is that the sites under palmitoyl-CoA control are different in microbial and animal systems.

I am unaware of any evidence for rapidly operating control mechanisms which directly effect the activity of animal fatty acid synthetases.   Instead, as we have seen, short-term control appears to be exerted primarily on Phase I enzymes, i.e., acetyl-CoA carboxylase and perhaps other lipogenic enzymes.   Whatever changes occur in the net capacity of hepatic or adipose tissue fatty acid synthetases reflect enzyme induction or derepression, the more delayed response of protein synthesis to external stimuli.   The rise or decline of enzyme levels in the wake of starvation, refeeding of carbohydrate or high fat diets, alloxan diabetes, and administration of insulin are impressive in magnitude and illustrate the vast capacity of the protein synthesis machinery to adjust to varying nutritional and hormonal states.   As previously noted, the lipogenic Phase I enzymes (acetyl-CoA carboxylase, ATP-citrate lyase and the various NADPH producers) are also regulated by induction and repression of protein synthesis (10).   Moreover, the inducing conditions, but not necessarily the immediate inducer signals for these lipogenic enzymes and for hepatic fatty acid synthetases seem to be the same.   Thus, to some extent at least the long-term adaptive response of the various target enzymes is coordinated and it may well turn out that the events occurring at multiple enzyme sites are synchronized as well.   The complexity of this regulatory network is, however, such as to discourage any assessment of the relative significance of each of the contributing mechanisms in the overall control of fatty acid synthesis.

I have previously noted the minimal impact of basic lipid research on chemotherapeutic approaches to atherosclerosis. In order to close on a hopeful and somewhat more positive note, I would
like to call attention to three substances which interfere with
specific events in lipid biosynthesis and do so by well understood
mechanisms, 3-Decynoyl-N-acetyl-cysteamine, developed in our laboratory as a substrate analogue, has been shown to block the formation
of unsaturated fatty acids in certain bacteria in a highly specific
manner (2).   The compound itself is not an inhibitor but a pseudo-
substrate, converted by the target enzyme into the allenic isomer,
2,3-decadienoyl-N-acetyl-cysteamine. This isomer in turn attaches
covalently to the active enzyme site and thereby causes irreversible inactivation.   3-Decynoyl-NAC is useful in a limited way as
an antibacterial agent and also for studying lipid-associated membrane phenomena.   But its main virtue is that it has led to the
discovery of a novel principle of enzyme inhibition.   This might
be described as "Enzyme Suicide" or the Trojan Horse effect.   Several other enzyme inhibitors acting in the same manner have since
been developed raising hopes that this general approach will be of
more than academic interest.

A naturally occurring lipid antimetabolite of great potential
called Cerulenin has recently been discovered by Omura et al. (13).
The antibiotic inhibits fatty acid synthetases of every type and
source by irreversible blockade of the enzyme that catalyzes the
condensation between acyl thioester and malonyl thioester in the
chain-lengthening process (22).   Cerulenin appears to interfere
also with an early step in cholesterol biosynthesis but it does
not effect other metabolic pathways.   A fairly specific antilipogenic agent, Cerulenin has a variety of interesting uses but its
clinical value is still untested.   Hopefully it will not join the
many promising yet toxic enzyme inhibitors which have disappeared
in the graveyard of forgotten wonder drugs.

Still another way of disrupting a metabolic pathway is illustrated by the mode of action of bacitracin.   In bacterial metabolism the antibiotic interferes with the regeneration of the polyisoprenoid lipid carrier which is essential for the biosynthesis
of the bacterial cell wall (18).   Bacitracin blocks squalene and
sterol synthesis in animal tissues similarly by complexing terpenoid
pyrophosphate intermediates.   Sequestering of substrate rather than
enzyme inhibition is the basis of this interesting type of metabolic
blockade.   The well-known toxicity of bacitracin may, of course, pre-
clude the use of this particular antibiotic as a hypocholesteremic
agent.   Whether there are useful lessons to be learned from the examples I have cited remains to be seen.   In any event, there are
now available several specific antilipogenic agents of known mode
of action and at the very least this knowledge should broaden our
understanding of lipid metabolism and its control.

Finally, I would like to share with you certain thoughts on

atherosclerosis research in general which I am sure are by no means original but which deserve perhaps to be reemphasized. It seems first of all that one major barrier to applying our basic know- ledge to the practical problem is the lack of a suitable animal model or at least the lack of assurance that the animal model is relevant. We may ask, for example, how significant for the human situation is the striking circadian pattern of HMG-CoA reductase in the rat and is it possible to obtain the answer experimentally? Is this and related phenomena attributable to the fact that rats are night feeders and consume their daily ration quickly in a single meal? By extension, has sufficient attention been paid to human food intake patterns in which the variables are not only diet quality but also the frequency and schedule of the daily meals? Is there any relation between life or work styles and atherosclero- sis? Is the pleasant habit of a postprandial siesta a factor in the relatively low incidence of atherosclerosis in Mediterranean countries?

Recently, four British scientists, nutritionists and physio- logists made the rather startling statement that the energy re- quirements of man and the balance of energy intake and expenditure are not known (4). They assert that the 30% of the world's po- pulation who have what is called an adequate food intake are real- ly eating too much and that an unknown proportion of the rest is really not undernourished. Illustrating the scope of the problem or perhaps our ignorance of human nutrition they further state that "in any group of 20 or more subjects with similar attributes and activities food intake can vary as much as two-fold; that some people, perhaps through some mechanism of adaptation are able to be healthy and active on energy intakes which by current standards would be regarded as inadequate; while other subjects can be given large quantities of additional food with little or no increase in body weight".

If we add to these uncertainties the current controversy about human vitamin requirements, both minimal and optimal, we come to realize how much research in human nutrition is still needed. To obtain the necessary information will be difficult not for technical reasons but because there are inherent and inviolate limitations to experimentation with humans.

What we can do, however, with little or no risk and for that matter without any expense is to listen to the advice given over the ages by men of wisdom. In his discourse on the "Art of Living Long" written at the age of 90, the 16th century Venetian Luigi Cornaro admonishes the reader:

"Il non saziarsi del tutto è il segreto della buona salute"
"Not to satiate one's self with food is the key and secret
  to health"

Can much better advice be given to-day?

REFERENCES

1. Bhavnani, B.R. and Short, R.V.
   Endocrinology 92: 657, 1973.
2. Bloch, K.
   Accts. of Chem. Res. 2: 193, 1969.
3. Clinkenbeard, K.D., Sugiyanne, T., Moss,J. and Lane, M.D.
   J. Biol. Chem. 248: 2275, 1973.
4. Durin, J.V.G.A., Edholm, O.G., Miller, D.S. and Waterlow, J.C.
   Nature 242: 418, 1973.
5. Edwards, P.E.
   J. Biol. Chem. 248: 2912, 1973.
6. Flick P. and Bloch, K.
   Unpublished.
7. Gould, R.G., Taylor, C.B., Hagerman, J.S., Warner,I. and
   Campbell, D.J.
   J. Biol. Chem. 201: 519, 1953.
8. Kandutsch, A.A. and Saucier, S.E.
   J. Biol. Chem. 244: 2299, 1969.
9. Knoche, H., Esders, T.W., Koths, K. and Bloch, K.
   J. Biol. Chem. 248: 2317, 1973.
10. Lowenstein, J.M.
    Handbook of Physiology-Endocrinology I: 415, 1971.
11. Lust, G and Lynen, F.
    Eur. J. Biochem. 7: 68, 1968.
12. Machida, Y., Bergeron, R., Flick, P. and Bloch, K.
    J. Biol. Chem. 248: 6246, 1973.
13. Omura, S., Katagiri, M., Nakagawa, A., Sano, S.,
    Nomura, S. and Hata, T.
    J. Antibiotics, Ser. A 20: 349, 1967.
14. Ono, T. and Bloch, K.
    Unpublished.
15. Ritter, M.C. and Dempsey, M.E.
    J. Biol. Chem. 246: 1536, 1971.
16. Scallen, T.J., Schuster, M.W. and Dtter, A.K.
    J. Biol. Chem. 246: 224, 1971.
17. Siperstein, M.D. and Fagan, V.M.
    Adv. Enzyme Regulation 2: 249, 1964.
18. Stone, K.J. and Strominger, J.L.
    Proc. Nat'l. Acad. Sci. (U.S.A.) 69: 1287, 1972.
19. Sumper, M. and Träuble, H.
    FEBS Letters 30: 29, 1973.
20. Tai, H.H. and Bloch, K.
    J. Biol. Chem. 247: 3767, 1972.
21. Taketa, K. and Pogell, B.M.
    J. Biol. Chem. 241: 720, 1966.
22. Vance, D., Goldberg, I., Mitsuhashi, O., Bloch, K.,
    Omura, S. and Nomura S.
    Biochem. Biophys. Res. Comm. 48: 649, 1972.
23. Volpe, J.J. and Vagelos, P.R.
    Ann. Rev. of Biochemistry 42: 21, 1973.

THE RELATIONSHIP OF DIET AND ATHEROSCLEROSIS

IN DIABETIC <u>MACACA</u> <u>NIGRA</u>

Charles F. Howard Jr.
Nutrition and Metabolic Diseases
Oregon Regional Primate Research Center
Beaverton, Oregon 97005 U.S.A.

Any possibility of gaining a clear view of the relationship between dietary carbohydrate and atherosclerosis depends upon clarification of the numerous metabolic events that interrelate carbohydrate management, insulin, and blood lipids; aberrations are reflected in obesity, coronary heart disease, and atherosclerosis. The ability to deal effectively with these various metabolic factors is hampered by not knowing which events are primary and which are secondary. Central to maintaining balanced glucose and lipid metabolism appears to be the capacity to produce, secrete, and utilize insulin. The defects in insulin control that accompany diabetes mellitus are apparent in hyperglycemia, glucose intolerance, and increased blood lipids. The last arises both because of the increased amount of carbohydrate available for lipid synthesis and because of the deranged lipid metabolism that stems from insulin abnormalities. The development of atherosclerotic lesions depends upon both <u>in</u> <u>situ</u> metabolism and external constituents in the blood. The role of insulin in this development may represent an anomaly in lesion development: on the one hand, excessive insulin can increase lipogenesis and other anabolic processes within the aorta; on the other, insulin deficiency could lead to changes in aortic metabolism as well as to increased blood glucose and lipids which further encourage the development of aortic lesions.

Cardiovascular complications and atherosclerosis are more prevalent in diabetic than in nondiabetic human beings (1-4). In this report on monkeys with a high percentage of spontaneous diabetes mellitus, I present preliminary data which relate the dietary regimen and clinical history of these animals to the eventual development of atherosclerosis. Although the number of

13

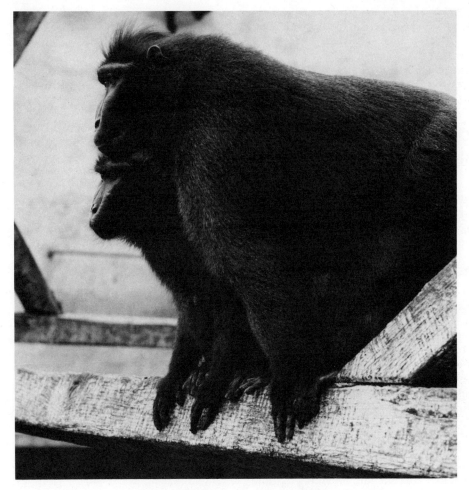

Fig. 1. Celebes black apes (<u>Macaca</u> <u>nigra</u>) with the
dominant male and one of the breeding females

experimental animals is not yet significantly large to establish an
absolute correlation between the appearance of atherosclerosis and
their previous clinical history of diabetes, the incidence of
aortic involvement in sudanophilia, fatty streak formation, and
overt lesions has been uniformly higher in monkeys with a diabetic
history than in their normal counterparts.

<u>Macaca</u> <u>nigra</u> (Celebes black apes) (Fig. 1) have a species-
specific diabetic syndrome (5) that is manifested in abnormal oral
and intravenous glucose tolerance tests (IV-GTT), impaired insulin
response to an IV-GTT, less insulin in serum taken after an overnight fast, hyperglycemia, hypertriglyceridemia, hyperprebetalipoproteinemia, and increased nonesterified fatty acids. Cholesterol

concentrations are generally low (<200 mg/dl) and do not correlate
with the diabetic status. Diabetic signs have been found among
many of the more than 55 Macaca nigra examined over the past few
years at the Oregon Primate Center as well as among the 23 members
of the Celebes colony at the Yerkes Primate Center, Atlanta, Georgia,
and among those available for clinical and necropsy studies from
several zoos. For the most part, the familial relationships of
these monkeys from various locations are unknown except that they
are from the Celebes Island (6). The working hypothesis is that prolonged inbreeding of this species within a small geographical sector
of this island has produced a diabetic syndrome that is hereditary
(Fig. 2). For example, some of the most recently purchased monkeys
tested only a month or so after leaving the Celebes Island show
impaired tolerance to an IV-GTT. The development of manifestations
secondary to genetic weakness should be further exacerbated over a
period of time by changes in their environment, particularly the
consumption of alien diets, in this case commercial chow pellets.

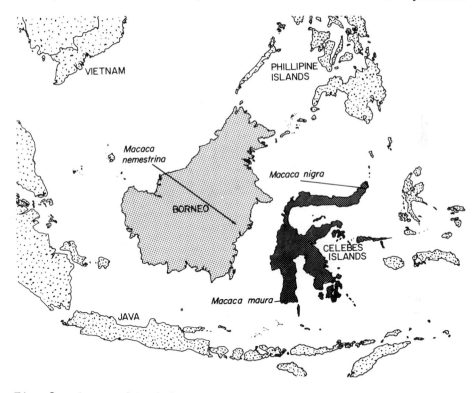

Fig. 2. Geographical location of Celebes Island showing the
  small sector from which Macaca nigra are obtained. A different
  species (6), Macaca maura, is indigenous to the southwest
  sector of the main island. Also indicated is Borneo where
  Macaca nemestrina, the most likely evolutionary ancestors of
  both species, are found.

All of the monkeys at the Oregon Primate Center receive Purina chow diet plus a daily supplement of fruit. Monkeys at other geographical locations within the United States receive either Purina chow or Wayne chow with fruit supplementation. The Purina chow diet contains 25% protein, 5 to 6% lipid, and approximately 55% carbohydrate, mainly in the form of starch. Analyses of the lipids show that triglyceride constitutes about 2.5% and cholesterol <0.01% of the total chow diet.

The genetic defect expressed in the diabetic syndrome (impaired insulin response, glucose mismanagement, elevated blood lipids), coupled with further impairments imposed by diet, should provide a milieu for the development of atherosclerosis. In the following, we will examine some of these interrelationships in Macaca nigra.

The data in Fig. 3 are compiled from 18 mature Macaca nigra, 9 to 20+ years of age, both living and dead. These animals become sexually mature at about 4-1/2 to 5-1/2 years; thus the ages covered in the figure correspond approximately to those of mature human beings between 30 and 60+ years of age. Juvenile diabetes at about 4 to 6 years of age has been found, but generally only insulin and glucose management are impaired; lipid

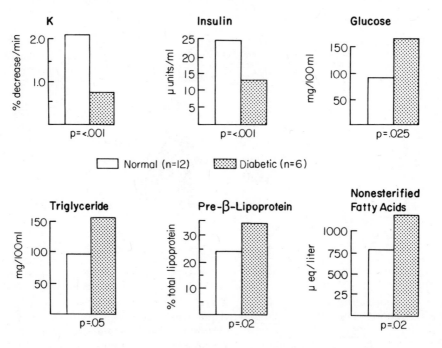

Fig. 3. Comparison of serum constituents in diabetic and normal Macaca nigra

concentrations remain low. Figure 3 shows 12 normal and 6 diabetic
monkeys with males and females present in both categories. Individual measurements for each monkey represent at least 2 to 5
separate analyses taken over a period of several years. Statistically significant differences exist between the diabetic and nondiabetic monkeys in all of the parameters examined. K* measures
the ability to clear glucose in an IV-GT (7). An individual K value
of about 1.7 or greater indicates a rapid clearance of glucose
whereas a K less than 1.0 indicates obvious impairment. Similar-
ities between these and human K values reflect the usefulness of
this mathematical equation for measuring quantitative glucose
management. Borderline diabetics (not included in Fig. 3) had K
values intermediate between the diabetic and nondiabetic categories,
and their clinical history showed varied responses in insulin,
glucose, and serum lipids. The significant K differences between
the two categories were due to the differences in insulin (immuno-
reactive insulin = IRI) response during the IV-GTT; a response of
rapid and sufficient quantities of IRI caused rapid glucose clearance which yielded Ks of 1.7 or greater, whereas a delay in the
amount or time of insulin secretion caused significantly less
clearance and low K values.

Glucose concentrations in the serum of fasted monkeys correlated inversely with the IRI, i.e., diabetic monkeys with less IRI
had greater glucose and the reverse was found in normal monkeys.
Similarly, increased triglyceride, prebetalipoprotein (measured on
agarose gel), and nonesterified fatty acids in the serum of diabetic monkeys had a statistically significant, inverse correlation
with the IRI. As a result, the aortas of these diabetic monkeys
were continuously exposed to blood that contained excess glucose
and lipids with much less insulin.

The reduction in insulin concentrations appears to be due to
a loss in beta cell reservoir and secretory capacity. Figure 4A
shows a normal isle of Langerhans; in Fig. 4B aldehyde-fuchsin stain
is used to visualize beta (insulin) granules within the beta cells.
Amyloid infiltration was seen in the isles of Langerhans, the
greatest infiltration being found in those monkeys with the most
severe clinical diabetes mellitus. Figure 4C shows the complete
loss of cells from an isle of Langerhans caused by amyloid infiltration. All the monkeys that had a clinical diabetic or borderline
diabetic state before death showed amyloid infiltration of the isles
of Langerhans in the pancreas; this was present in those monkeys
from Oregon as well as those from the Yerkes Primate Center and from
zoos. Whether this phenomenon is a primary event that leads
to the necrosis of the beta and alpha cells or whether it is
secondary to their necrosis is not known. The net result is the

$$*K = \frac{0.693 \times 100}{t_{1/2}} \text{ \% decrease of serum glucose per minute.}$$

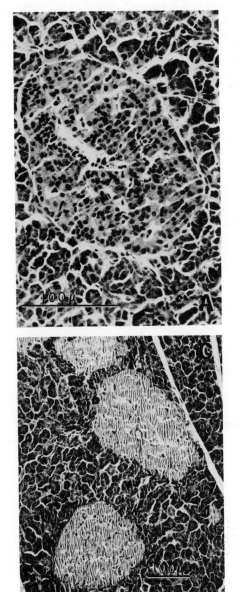

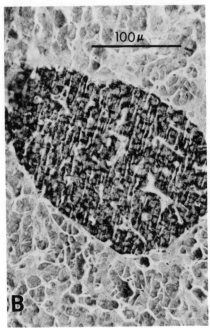

Fig. 4A. Normal pancreatic isle of Langerhans (hematoxylin and eosin - H & E).

4B. Normal pancreatic isle of Langerhans showing insulin granules in the beta cells (aldehyde-fuchsin trichrome).

4C. Amyloid infiltration into isles of Langerhans of diabetic monkeys (sulfated alcian blue).

same: diminution in the reservoir of available insulin. With the progressive loss of beta cells over a long period of time, the ability of the monkey to maintain homeostasis is impaired, and progressively increased concentrations of blood glucose and lipids result. Apparently there is a close correlation between the degree and severity of atherosclerosis and the functional appearance of the isles of Langerhans. Usually the degeneration of the islet tissue was reflected in the clinical history although an occasional

Table 1. Clinical and necropsy information on Macaca nigra

Diabetic class and age*	K**	Insulin (μunits/ml)	Glucose (mg/100 ml)	Triglycerides (mg/100 ml)	Prebeta-lipoprotein (%)	Isles of Langerhans histology	Aortic involvement
Aged normal monkeys (4)	1.81	20.9	109	124	17.6	Normal to 30%	10-50% sudanophilic blush; 5-15% roughened streaks; few, small discrete lesions
Aged diabetic monkeys (3)	0.40	10.5	160	176	>30	Complete amyloidosis	>75% sudanophilic blush; lesions—ranged from minimal involvement at intercostals, renals, etc., up to 85% of surface in fibrous, lipid lesions
Juvenile diabetic monkeys (2)	0.56	12.0	107	113	13.2	50% loss of beta granules; cells normal	Aortas with no sudanophilia or lesion involvement

*Aged is 15 to 20 years, juvenile 4 to 5 years; number of monkeys is given in parentheses.

**$K = \dfrac{0.693 \times 100}{t_{1/2}}$ % decrease per minute where $t_{1/2}$ is the time required for the blood glucose concentration to decrease by half during an intravenous glucose tolerance test.

autopsy revealed some loss of islet capacity that was not identified earlier. Atherosclerosis is present in those monkeys with
morphological changes in the isles of Langerhans to a varied extent;
failure to detect clinical diabetes does not rule out the subtle
effects of the loss of the secretory capacity of beta cell insulin
to alter metabolism sufficiently to produce some aortic involvement.
A few living monkeys have hyperinsulinemia or an adequate secretion
of insulin with impaired K values and increased lipids, but these
are not common.

     Clinical and necropsy data on aged normal, aged diabetic, and
juvenile diabetic monkeys are summarized in Table 1. Since age is
a major factor in the development of atherosclerosis, the two
major groups of monkeys compared in Table 1 range from 15 to 20
years old; an approximate comparable age of human beings would be
from 45 or 50 to about 60+ years of age. When these two groups
are compared, the effects of age are minimized. The same general
comparisons presented in Fig. 3 can be seen in these data, though
there is not yet enough data for statistical analyses. Glucose
clearance during an IV-GTT is impaired in aged diabetics. This is
related to the lower quantities of insulin as are the increased
glucose, triglyceride, and prebetalipoprotein concentrations in the
aged diabetic monkeys. The clinical data on the two juvenile diabetic monkeys show the impaired IV-GTT related to lower concentrations of insulin in response to the glucose stress of the test. The
fasted glucose, triglycerides, and prebetalipoproteins during
normal conditions are all at or below those levels found in the
aged, normal Macaca nigra.

     Histologically, the architecture of the isles of Langerhans
among the four aged nondiabetic monkeys was normal or ranged up to
about 30% loss of beta cells. In the aged diabetic, amyloid infiltration was extreme with almost complete loss of identifiable cells.
In the juvenile diabetics, the general architecture of the isles of
Langerhans appeared normal with hematoxylin and eosin stain but
differential stains revealed at least 50% loss of beta granules.
Both of the juvenile diabetic monkeys died suddenly after an
apparently rapid onset and loss of ability to manage glucose
properly.

     The extent of aortic involvement represented a spectrum for
the normal and for the diabetic aged monkeys. The normal monkeys
ranged from moderate to about 50% sudanophilic blush and some contained roughened streaks and a few small discrete lesions. Of the
three aged diabetic monkeys, the one with the least involvement had
greater than 75% sudanophilia and numerous lesions at the intercostal and renal arteries and in the arch. The other two had extensive lesion involvement of the aorta which covered 65 to 85% of
the surface. The aortas of the juvenile diabetics were clear and
free of any atherosclerotic involvement. The most logical

assumption is that in the juvenile diabetics the impairment in glucose management and any concomitant changes in blood lipids were not present long enough to aggravate the development of athero-sclerosis. Thus the age factor does seem to be of importance in these monkeys since atherosclerosis was not present in the juvenile diabetics but did appear in some aged normal as well as all aged diabetic monkeys.

The aorta from one of the juvenile diabetic monkeys age 4-1/2 years is shown in Fig. 5. Clinical history showed a marked loss in the ability to respond to an IV-GTT and less fasted IRI although fasted glucose, triglyceride, and prebetalipoprotein concentra-tions were normal. At necropsy the pancreas beta cells appeared normal but contained only about half the normal complement of beta granules. The glucose mismanagement and lack of lipid increases were probably minimal and lasted for such a short period of time that no sudanophilia or lesions appeared in the aorta. Some medial

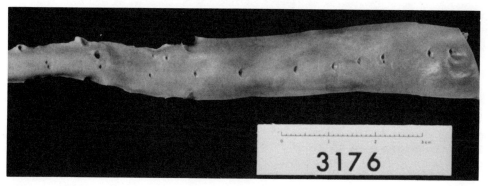

Fig. 5. Aorta from juvenile monkey who died shortly after the onset of the diabetic syndrome. All aortas pictured in Fig. 5 through 9 were fixed in formalin and then stained with Sudan IV.

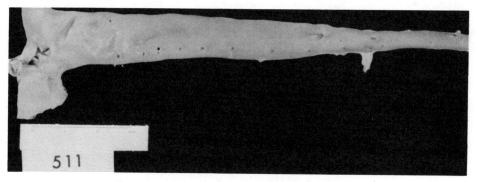

Fig. 6. Normal aorta from aged female

thickening was to be expected by this age, but the intima and media appeared normal.

The artery of an aged female monkey with a completely normal clinical history throughout her life span is shown in Fig. 6. The aorta is slightly thickened and has a sudanophilic blush over 40 to 50% of the intimal surface; no raised lesions or fatty streaks are visible in this aorta. Examination of the pancreatic isles of Langerhans revealed normal architecture. This was the best example of a normal aorta with a normal clinical history; the other three normal monkeys had somewhat more aortic involvement. The aorta pictured in Fig. 7 represents involved aorta among the more normal

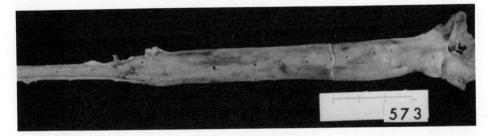

Fig. 7. Aorta from a monkey classed as normal but which
had occasional hyperglycemia and some loss of beta
cells in the isles of Langerhans

monkeys. There is an overall average of about 30 to 40% sudano-philia, approximately 15 to 20% raised fatty streaks, some roughened areas, and a few small discrete lesions in the arch. This particular monkey had a normal IV-GTT and adequate IRI, but necropsy showed about a 30% loss of the beta cells of the isles of Langerhans. Aortas from the other two monkeys categorized as clinically normal had 10 to 30% sudanophilic blush, 5 to 25% of raised roughened areas and streaks, but only a few small discrete lesions. The pancreatic isles of Langerhans had some beta granule loss in one case and 40% loss of beta cells in the other.

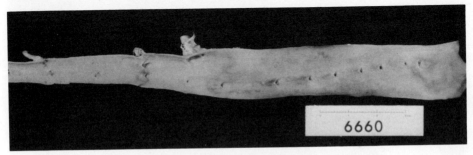

Fig. 8. Aorta with the least involvement
among the diabetic monkeys

The aorta with the least involvement from among the three
diabetic aged monkeys is pictured in Fig. 8.   This monkey was a
gift from the Oklahoma City Zoo where diabetes had been diagnosed.
Some clinical studies had been done before its arrival in Oregon;
only limited studies could be done before it died.   The IV-GTT K
was 0.49 and the fasting IRI was 10.5 units/mg.   There was hyperglycemia (200 to 300 mg/100 ml), and the prebetalipoprotein
concentration run on a blood sample taken shortly before death
revealed 62% of the lipoprotein present as prebetalipoprotein.   How
long it had had a clinical history of diabetes is not known.
Certainly the severity of the aorta pictured in Fig. 8 would be
somewhat greater than that found at the upper limit of the normal
aged monkeys (Fig. 7).   The aorta in Fig. 8 had about a 75% sudanophilic blush and a significant number of raised lesions at the
intercostal and renal arteries.   It was generally thickened and
there was evidence of roughening and some possible fatty streaks.
There was complete amyloidosis of the isles of Langerhans in the
pancreas of this monkey.

The aorta pictured in Fig. 9 is from a severely diabetic
Macaca nigra studied over an 8-year period of time at the Oregon

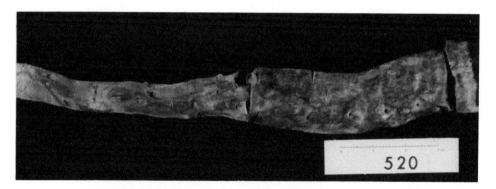

Fig. 9.   Extensive involvement of an aorta
from a severely diabetic Macaca nigra

Primate Center.   Clinical history revealed abnormal IV-GTT,
minimal amounts of IRI, and increased concentrations of fasted
blood glucose, triglycerides, and prebetalipoprotein.   At necropsy,
the pancreas showed complete infiltration by amyloid material
(Fig. 4C) into the isles of Langerhans.   The aortic surface
had some 60% of the surface involved in fatty streaks and lesions.
The third diabetic monkey was a gift of the Denver Zoo (Colorado)
and was judged to be about the same age as this severely diabetic
monkey.   What little clinical history was available before its
death indicated a severe diabetic condition, and the involvement
of the aorta was comparable to that pictured in Fig. 9.

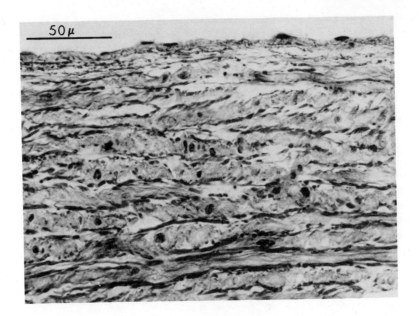

Fig. 10. Normal intima and media from a
clinically normal monkey (H & E)

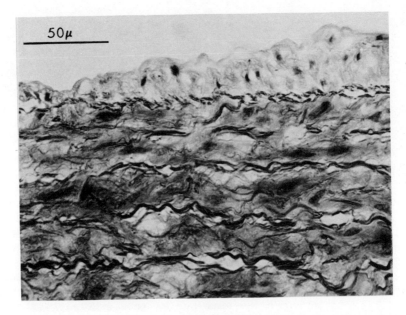

Fig. 11. Slight intimal thickening in an aorta from a monkey
that was generally normal clinically (H & E)

Histological examination of aortic sections showed many of the changes expected with the onset and progression of athero- sclerosis. The histological section in Fig. 10 from the aorta of this normal, aged monkey pictured macroscopically in Fig. 6 shows minimal intima and normal appearing media. Figure 11 shows the aorta from a monkey generally normal in clinical measurements but with occasional indications of inability to respond to an IV-GTT; the isles of Langerhans appeared normal. Some replication and extension of intimal cells is seen in Fig. 11 but the internal elastic lamina is still intact.

Figure 12 presents a section of lesion from a diabetic monkey. Increased intimal thickening and proliferation of cells and sub-

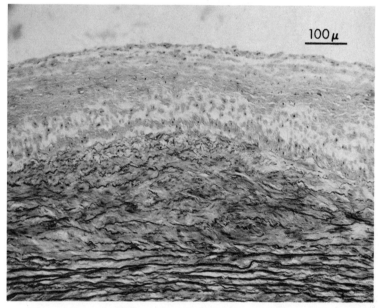

Fig. 12.   Lesion from a diabetic monkey (H & E)

intimal disorganization of the media can be seen. A higher magni- fication of a lesion from a diabetic monkey (Fig. 13) shows the extent of vacuolization, foam cells, and lesion development. The sulfated alcian blue stain revealed no amyloid infiltration into the aorta as there was in the isles of Langerhans in this monkey. Elastic fibers are present near the base of the lesion and can also be seen throughout the lesion (Fig. 14) in addition to lipid deposition. Results similar to those shown in Fig. 12-14 were seen when sections were taken through lesions of less diabetic or of normal monkeys with a minimum number of lesions.

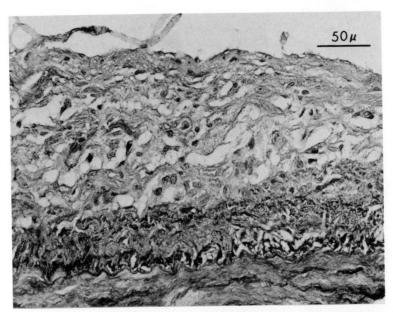

Fig. 13. Aortic lesion from a diabetic monkey stained
for possible infiltration of amyloid-like material
(sulfated alcian blue)

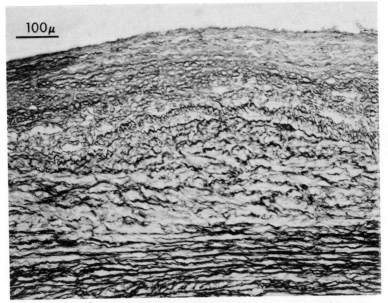

Fig. 14. Aortic lesion stained to visualize
elastin fibers (orcein)

When sections were stained with Sudan IV, some darker areas were apparent. In Fig. 15, in addition to staining preferentially for fat, Nomarski differential interference-contrast microscopy was used. The darkest areas contain lipid and appear raised

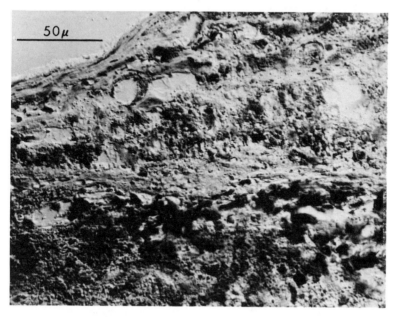

Fig. 15. Aortic lesion stained to visualize lipid
deposits and viewed with Nomarski differential
interference-contrast optics (Sudan IV)

whereas the vacuoles are clear and appear as a depressed background. This section is only through the intimal lesion area and does not extend into the media. Considering that this aorta had been previously stained for sudanophilia grossly, the residual lipid still present to stain histologically indicates that a greater amount was probably present initially.

Crystalline clefts, presumably cholesterol, were seen in lesions of the severely diabetic as well as in a lesion of a normal monkey. These are visualized in Fig. 16. The Sudan IV stain shows darker areas of lipid deposition in the intimal lesion and crystalline structures in the subintimal area. With Nomarski optics, the enlargement area pictured in Fig. 17 shows a distinct prismatic crystal as well as sheaves of needle-like crystalline structures.

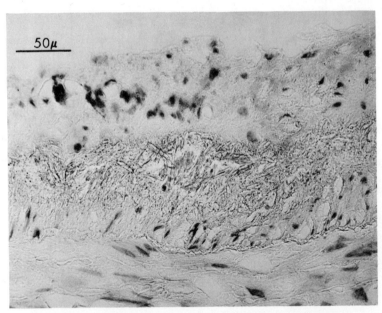

Fig. 16. Lesion showing lipid staining material and presence
of crystalline formations (Sudan IV, normal optics)

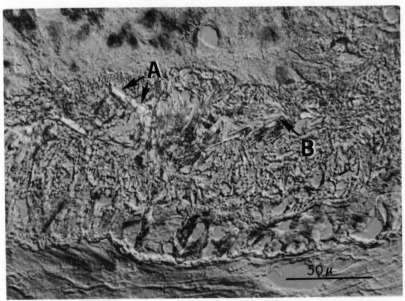

Fig. 17. Enlarged area of Fig. 16 using Nomarski optics. A
prismatic crystal is seen at A and one of several sheaves
of needle-like bundles of crystals is at B (Sudan IV)

The extent of atherosclerosis in these monkeys is related to their age and to their diabetic status during life. Even among those aged monkeys that appear clinically normal, there are some changes in glucose management, blood lipids, and pancreatic histology. Often with apparently only slight deviations from the clinically normal state, there is a greater tendency towards aortic sudanophilia, raised roughened streaks, and occasional small lesions. The spectrum of aortic involvement reflects the clinical history and pancreatic histology. Normal aged Macaca nigra have much less tendency towards atherosclerosis than those with a diabetic history. The diabetic monkeys have greater aortic involvement of sudanophilia as well as greater medial thickening, fatty raised streaks, and extensive lesion development. The least involved among aortas from diabetic monkeys is still greater than normal aortas; the diabetic aortas show further severe involvement which relates to their clinical history and isles of Langerhans pathology. Thus even with the small number of samples present, there is a distinct correlation between inability to effectively deal metabolically with glucose and lipids and the extent of atherosclerosis, exclusive of the age of the monkey.

These Macaca nigra are maintained on much the same kind of diet as are other monkey species at the Oregon Primate Center and in most other institutions, yet other species apparently do not develop the diabetic syndrome. There have been several reports of spontaneous atherosclerosis in nonhuman primates that were not challenged with atherogenic diets (8-14). Carbohydrate intolerance and possible diabetes were reported in squirrel monkeys (15) some of which also exhibited atherosclerosis. However, this report directly relates the degree and severity of atherosclerosis to the intensity of the clinical syndrome of diabetes mellitus in each of the monkeys.

Obviously, the Macaca nigra cannot adequately handle the glucose load that is presented to them in this diet. The 55% carbohydrate content is probably a greater insult than the 5 to 6% lipid concentration. The fatty acids of the chow are 70% mono- and diunsaturated and the triglycerides of the serum contain about 2/3 of the fatty acids present in an unsaturated form. The cholesterol content $\leq 0.01\%$ is far less than that in atherogenic diets. Thus, there is little likelihood that the lipid constitutes a major atherogenic insult. Increased blood lipid concentrations must therefore arise primarily from endogenous sources. Increased blood glucose and lipid concentrations constitute minimal to severe insult to the aorta over a prolonged period of time and result in the typical manifestations of atherosclerosis.

Diet probably plays a secondary role to the primary metabolic
aberration, insulin production. Impairment within the monkey to
secrete adequate, functional quantities of insulin undoubtedly lies
at the root of most of its inability to adequately control glucose
and to maintain normal concentrations of lipids in the blood.
Metabolic abnormalities arise because of decreasing reservoirs of
insulin secretory capacity in the beta cells. Thus, in the Macaca
nigra, there is a direct link between their inability to handle the
carbohydrate in their diet, which stems from insulin insufficiency,
and the manifestations of the diabetic syndrome which create
enough metabolic abberrations to cause increased aortic atherosclerosis.

ACKNOWLEDGMENTS

I thank JoAnn Wolff and Lynne Bonnett for their fine technical
assistance. This research was supported by U.S. Public Health
Service Grants No. RR-00163 and No. HE-09744 and by grants from
the Kroc Foundation and the Medical Research Foundation of Oregon.
This is Publication No. 685 from the Oregon Regional Primate
Research Center.

SELECTED REFERENCES

1. Clawson, B. J., and Bell, E. T. Incidence of fatal coronary
   disease in nondiabetic and in diabetic persons. Arch. Path.
   48: 105-106, 1949.
2. Liebow, I. M., Hellerstein, H. K., and Miller, M.
   Arteriosclerotic heart disease in diabetes mellitus.
   Am. J. Med. 18: 438-447, 1955.
3. Robertson, W. B., and Strong, J. P. Atherosclerosis in persons with hypertension and diabetes mellitus. Lab. Invest.
   18: 538-551, 1968.
4. Bradley, R. F. Cardiovascular diseases. In Joslin's
   Diabetes Mellitus, Marble, A., White, P., Bradley, R. F.,
   and Krall, L. P., eds. Lea and Febiger, Philadelphia, 1971,
   pp 417-477.
5. Howard, C. F. Jr. Spontaneous diabetes in Macaca nigra.
   Diabetes 21: 1077-1090, 1972.
6. Fooden, J. Taxonomy and evolution of the monkeys of the
   Celebes. Bibliotheca Primatologia, No. 10, Karger, Basel,
   1969.
7. Lundbaek, K. Intravenous glucose tolerance as a tool in the
   definition and diagnosis of diabetes mellitus. Brit. Med. J.
   1: 1507-1513, 1962.

8. Gillman, J., and Gilbert, C.   Atherosis in the baboon (Papio ursinus), its pathogenesis and etiology.   Exp. Med. Surg. 15: 181-221, 1957.
9. McGill, H. C. Jr., Strong, J. P., Holman, R. L., and Werthessen, N. T.   Arterial lesions in the Kenya baboon. Circ. Res. 8: 670-679, 1960.
10. Middleton, C. C., Clarkson, T. B., Lofland, H. B., and Prichard, R. W.   Atherosclerosis in the squirrel monkey. Arch. Pathol. 78: 16-23, 1964.
11. Clarkson, T. B.   Spontaneous atherosclerosis in subhuman primates.   In Comparative Atherosclerosis, Roberts, J. C. Jr., Strauss, R., and Cooper, M. S., eds.   Harper and Row, New York, 1965, pp 211-214.
12. Strong, J. P.   Arterial lesions in primates.   In Comparative Atherosclerosis, Roberts, J. C. Jr., Strauss, R., and Cooper, M. S., eds.   Harper and Row, New York, 1965, pp 244-252.
13. Malinow, M. R., and Maruffo, C. A.   Naturally occurring atherosclerosis in howler monkeys (Alouatta caraya).   J. Atheroscler. Res. 6: 368-380, 1966.
14. Andrus, S. B., Portman, O. W., and Riopelle, A. J.   Comparative studies of spontaneous and experimental atherosclerosis in primates.   II.   Lesions in chimpanzees including myocardial infarction and cerebral aneurysms.   Prog. Biochem. Pharm. 4: 393-419, 1968.
15. Davidson, I. W. F., Lang, C. M., and Blackwell, W. L. Impairment of carbohydrate metabolism of the squirrel monkey. Diabetes 16: 395-401, 1967.

THE EFFECTS OF PHYSICAL EXERCISE IN REVERSING

EXPERIMENTAL ATHEROSCLEROSIS

H.Y.C. WONG, S.N. DAVID, S.O. ORIMILIKWE, F.B. JOHNSON

Department of Physiology, Howard University
College of Medicine and Armed Forces Institute of
Pathology, Washington, D.C.

Two studies were performed in this experiment. Part 1, a group of cockerels was placed on plain mash while the others were on an atherogenic diet. Eight weeks later it was observed that the plasma cholesterol level of the cholesterol fed birds was increased ten fold when compared to the controls on plain mash. Several birds were sacrificed and no aortic atherosclerosis was observed in any of the controls on plain mash while all those on an atherogenic regimen had lesions averaging 2.1 (based on zero to four). Part 2, nine birds from each regimen were exercised while nine others served as controls. After eight weeks, it was found that exercise had no significant effect on body weight, plasma cholesterol or adrenal weights. The heart weights of the exercised groups on plain mash or a cholesterol diet were heavier than similarly fed sedentary groups. No aortic atherosclerosis was observed in any of the groups on plain mash. The non-exercised atherogenic fed birds had much more severe atherosclerosis than those exercised on the same regimen. The hydroxyproline concentration of collagen in the thoracic aorta was lowest in the exercised group on a cholesterol diet and was less than the exercised plain mash group. Physical activity had no effect on aortic elastin concentration. Exercise did not significantly alter the collagen to elastin ratio in the thoracic aortas of cockerels on plain mash, but it significantly lowered the C/E ratio of exercised birds on an atherogenic regimen. Our studies indicate that although moderate exercise had no effect on plasma cholesterol, it was capable of reversing aortic atherosclerosis in cockerels induced by and maintained on a high cholesterol diet. The decrease in aortic

33

atherosclerosis in the exercised group on an atherogenic regiman
(0.3) compared to a similarly fed sedentary group (2.9) may be
partially explained by the decrease in C/E ratio. It is generally
accepted that exercise results in reduced plasma cholesterol and
lower incidence and severity of aortic and coronary atherosclerosis
of cholesterol fed animals when compared to non-exercised sedentary groups. Although the specific mechanism by which stress or
physical activity seems to protect against aortic and coronary
atherosclerosis is obscure, several postulations have been offer-
ed. Mann et al (1955) reported that the caloric supply of young
men could be doubled and this did not result in an increase in
serum cholesterol so long as the surplus energy was expended as
heat and muscular energy. It was reported by Malinow et al (1968)
that physical activity is related to an apparent increase in the
oxidation of cholesterol in rats. They also obtained similar results from anesthesized rats and squirrel monkeys when they were
stimulated electrically (1968). In man, Malinow (1968) observed
that physical exercise resulted in an increase of the side chain
clevage of cholesterol. To our knowledge no report exists on the
effect of exercise on arterial wall connective tissue as related
to atherosclerosis. It has been reported by Fischer and Llaurado
(1966) that the combination of collagen and elastin comprise over
one-half the dry weight of the arterial wall. Fischer (1972) observed in rats without estrogen therapy, the concentration of arterial collagen was likely to be increased. This resulted in a
marked elevation of collagen to elastin ration which is an index
of the rigidity of a blood vessel. Burton (1954) suggested that
the passive tension of the wall is primarily due to collagen and
elastin. A low collagen to elastin ratio (C/E) increases the
distensibility in blood vessels like the aorta with high concentration of elastin fibers. Conversely, it was reported by Fischer
and Llaurado (1971) that the relatively stiff coronary artery has
a high proportion of collagen fibers and is inclined toward atherosclerosis. The present study was undertaken to determine whether
exercise could reverse atherosclerosis induced by and maintained
on an atherogenic diet, and the effect of stress upon the hydroxyproline concentration of collagen and elastin in aortas of cockerels
with atherosclerosis.

MATERIALS AND METHODS

This experiment was performed in two parts: Part one: One
hundred-twenty-four 50-week-old-Hy-line cockerels were divided
into two groups of 62 birds each. One group was maintained on
a commercial plain mash (P.M.) diet while the other group was fed
an atherogenic diet (A.D.) consisting of a mixture of P.M. plus
2% cholesterol and 5% cottonseed oil by weight. After fasting
overnight the body weight and plasma samples of all birds were

taken at the beginning of the experiment and every two weeks thereafter. Total plasma cholesterol was determined by the method of
Wong et al (1965). After eight weeks on these diets seven birds
from each group were sacrificed at random to determine the severity
of aortic atherosclerosis according to the procedure of Katz and
Stamler (1953). All birds on an atherogenic diet had aortic lesions while cockerels on plain mash had none. Part two: Nine birds
from each regimen were exercised while nine others served as controls. Groups thus were formed as follows: I. Controls, P.M.;
II. P.M. + exercise; III. A.D.; IV. A.D. + exercise. Exercise con-
sisted of running in a circular treadmill 20 minutes twice daily,
5 consecutive days a week at a rate of approximately 750 yards
daily. At the end of an additional eight weeks these cockerels
were sacrificed. The hearts, adrenals and thyroids were excised
and weighed. The aortae were rapidly removed, trimmed of extra-
neous tissue and opened longitudinally to be grossly graded by
the method mentioned above. The aortae were blotted with filter
paper and weighed. A section of the thoracic aorta was removed,
weighed and minced. The hydroxyproline concentration of collagen
and elastin was determined according to the method of Newman and
Logan (1950).

     The collagen content of the thoracic aorta was expressed in
mg/100 mg of dry, lipid-free aortic tissue. This was done by
using the factor of 7.46 to convert the values of hydroxyproline
into those of collagen. Elastin is expressed as mg of hydroxyproline liberated by hydroxylysis of this protein by 100 mg of
dry, lipid-free aorta. The amount of nitrogen in the collagen
extract was determined by the procedure of Houck and Jacob (1958).
Histological sections of the aorta and coronary arteries were made
and strained by the Oil-Red-O method (1968).

                              RESULTS

     Groups of cockerels fed plain mash or an atherogenic diet for
the first eight weeks of the experiment gained weight, but the
weight gains were not significantly different (Table I). Birds
were then randomly selected from the control groups on plain mash
or an atherogenic regimen for the experimental groups. Our results
indicate that exercise had no marked effect upon the body weight
of any of the groups. Table II summarizes the plasma cholesterol
levels of cockerels selected from plain mash or the atherogenic
diet prior to the beginning of the second part of the experiment.
There were no significant difference between the initial and final
plasma cholesterol values of the controls on plain mash. Birds fed
a cholesterol regimen showed a ten fold increase in plasma cholesterol by the end of the first eight weeks. The data indicated that
exercise had no effect on the plasma cholesterol of cockerels on
either plain mash or on a cholesterol diet. Prior to the second

Table I. Effect of Exercise on Body Weights of Cockerels with Induced Atherosclerosis

Groups	No. of Birds	Initial Wt. (g)	Final Wt. (g)
BEFORE EXPERIMENT			
Controls, plain mash (P.M.)	62	2079 $\pm$ 7°	2180 $\pm$ 9
Atherogenic diet (A.D.)°°	62	2089 $\pm$ 14	2188 $\pm$ 17
AFTER EXPERIMENT			
Controls, plain mash	9	2043 $\pm$ 53	2005 $\pm$ 89
P.M. + exercise°°°	9	2085 $\pm$ 60	2146 $\pm$ 62
Atherogenic diet (A.D.)	9	2107 $\pm$ 67	2109 $\pm$ 86
A.D. + exercise	9	2065 $\pm$ 31	2178 $\pm$ 35

° Standard error of mean
°° 2% cholesterol + 5% cottonseed oil added to mash
°°° 750 yds. daily, 5 days per week

Table II. Influence of Exercise on Plasma Cholesterol of Cockerels with Induced Atherosclerosis

Groups	No. of Birds	Initial mg/100ml	Final mg/100ml
BEFORE EXPERIMENT			
Controls, plain mash (P.M.)	7	92 ± 2°	95 ± 3
Atherogenic diet (A.D.)°°	7	90 ± 3	874 ± 206
AFTER EXPERIMENT			
Controls, plain mash	9	91 ± 3	93 ± 3
P.M. + exercise°°°	9	84 ± 3	87 ± 4
A.D.	9	1276 ± 173	1195 ± 154
A.D. + exercise	9	953 ± 34	906 ± 32

° Standard error of mean
°° 2% cholesterol + 5% cottonseed oil added to mash
°°° 750 yds. daily, 5 days per week

Table III. Effect of Exercise on Gross and Microscopic Grading of Aortic and Coronary Atherosclerosis

GROUPS	No. of Birds	Gross grading Aortic No. with lesions	%	Avg.	Microscopic grading Aortic No. with lesions	%	Coronary No. with lesions	%
BEFORE EXPERIMENT								
Controls, plain mash (P.M.)	7	0	0	0°°°				
Atherogenic diet (A.D.)°	7	7	100	2.1				
AFTER EXPERIMENT								
Controls, P.M.	9	0	0	0	0	0	0	0
P.M. + exercise°°	9	0	0	0	0	0	0	0
A.D.	9	9	100	2.9	9	100	7	78
A.D. + exercise	9	5	55	0.3	9	100	55	55

° 2% cholesterol + 5% cottonseed oil added to mash
°° 750 yds. daily, 5 days per week
°°° Based on zero to four

part of the experiment, no gross aortic lesions were observed in
any of the controls on plain mash while all birds on an atherogenic regimen had atherosclerosis with an average gross grading
of 2.1 on a scale of zero to four (Table III). After eight weeks
of exercise no lesions were noted in any of the controls on plain
mash.   In the group fed an atherogenic diet only, all cockerels
had aortic lesions with a grading of 2.9 which was much more severe than the 2.1 grading of a group of similarly fed birds before the second part of the experiment began. Five of nine birds
of the cholesterol fed group which were exercised had lesions
with an average grading of 0.3.   These findings were significantly lower than the 2.9 of the similarly fed non-exercised group.
It was also lower than the initial grading of 2.1 for the cholesterol fed group even though these birds were continued to be
fed a cholesterol rich diet for another eight weeks. No aortic
atherosclerosis was seen microscopically for cockerels on plain
mash whether exercised or not. All birds had microscopically ob-
servable lesions after being on an atherogenic regimen. The degree of atherosclerosis was significantly less for exercise birds
than for non-exercised birds. Neither exercised nor non-exercised cockerels on plain mash showed coronary lesions, while the
birds fed a cholesterol diet showed an increase in coronary lesions. For the group on an atherogenic regimen, seven of nine
birds had coronary lesions while for the similarly fed group which
was exercised, five of nine cockerels had lesions. Histologic
sections of the aortas of control cockerels, whether exercised or
not, showed no lipid deposition on the intima (Fig. 1 and 2).
The atherogenic fed cockerels evidenced marked increase of lipid
deposition on the intima, while a similar group on the same diet
which was exercised, little if any aortic atherosclerosis was observed (Fig. 3 and 4). No coronary lesions were observed in any
of the control groups (Fig. 5 and 6). Cockerels on an atherogenic
regimen showed coronary atherosclerosis (Fig. 7) while a similar
exercised group on the same diet, little if any, coronary lesions
were observed (Fig. 7 and 8). Table IV indicated that the heart
weights were not significantly different for cockerels on plain
mash or on an atherogenic regimen before the experiment began.
After eight weeks of exercise, however, it was observed that the
heart weight of the exercised groups on either plain mash or on a
cholesterol regimen were markedly greater than their non-exercised
controls (p < .05) and (p < .02) respectively. The weight of the
heart of the atherogenic diet group with exercise was significantly greater than the controls on plain mash (p < .01). Before the
experiment began, the adrenal and thyroid weights of the birds fed
either plain mash or on an atherogenic regimen were not statistically different. After exercising for eight weeks, our data indicate
that physical activity did not have a marked effect on either the
adrenal or thyroid weights of any of the exercised groups (Table V).
The adrenal glands of the atherogenic group with exercise were

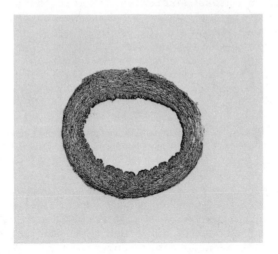

Fig. 1. Histologic section of aorta of controls on plain mash, no atherosclerosis is observed.   X 12

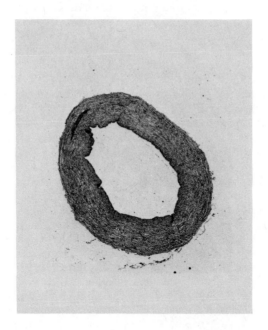

Fig. 2. Aorta of control, which was exercised, showing no atherosclerosis.   X 12

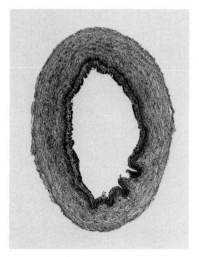

Fig. 3. Section of aorta of atherogenic fed cockerel showing lipid deposition in the intima.   X 12

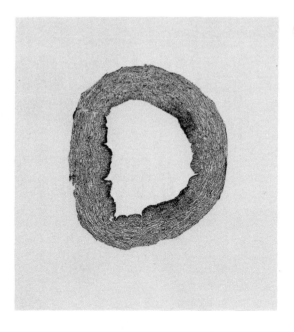

Fig. 4. Slight atherosclerosis is observed in aorta of atherogenic fed cockerel which was exercised.   X 12

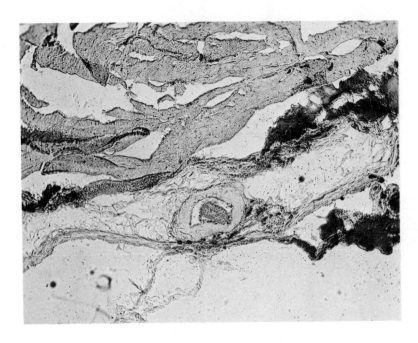

Fig. 5. Section of coronary artery of control on plain mash showing no atherosclerosis.   X 90

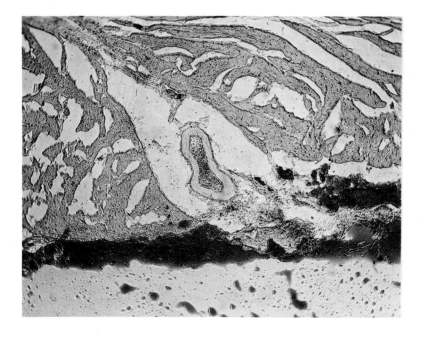

Fig. 6. Coronary artery of control on plain mash + exercise
showing no lesion.   X 90

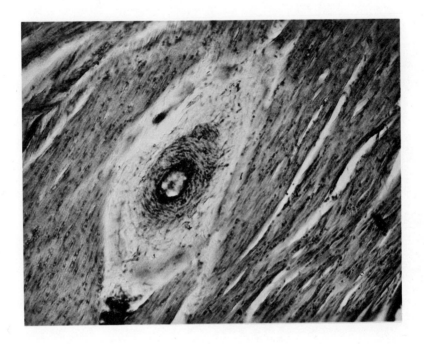

Fig. 7. Section of coronary artery of cockerel fed an atherogenic diet only depicting atherosclerosis of the intima.   X 90

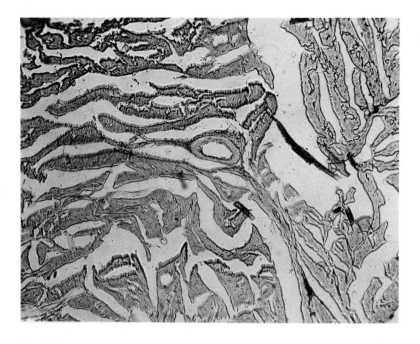

Fig. 8. Coronary artery of atherogenic cockerel which was exercised showing no lesion.   X 90

Table IV.   Changes in Heart Weights of Cockerels with Induced Atherosclerosis by Exercise

BEFORE EXPERIMENT

GROUPS	No. of Birds	Weight (g)
Controls, plain mash (P.M.)	7	11.9 ± .56°
Atherogenic diet (A.D.)°°	7	11.7 ± .49

AFTER EXPERIMENT

Controls, P.M.	9	10.2 ± .49
P.M. + exercise°°°	9	12.2 ± .61
A.D.	9	11.5 ± .46
A.D. + exercise	9	13.6 ± .51

° Standard error of mean
°° 2% cholesterol + 5% cottonseed oil added to mash
°°° 750 yds. daily, 5 days per week

p < .05 – Controls vs P.M. + exercise
p < .01 – Controls vs A.D. + exercise
p < .02 – A.D. vs A.D. + exercise

Table V. Influence of Exercise on Adrenal and Thyroid Weights of Cockerels with Induced Atherosclerosis

GROUPS	No. of Birds	Adrenal Wt. (mg)	Thyroid Wt. (mg)
BEFORE EXPERIMENT			
Controls, plain mash (P.M.)	7	205 ± 10°	215 ± 21
Atherogenic diet (A.D.)°°	7	222 ± 22	198 ± 29
AFTER EXPERIMENT			
Controls, P.M.	9	194 ± 11	200 ± 17
P.M. + exercise°°°	9	227 ± 16	187 ± 8
A.D.	9	233 ± 12	247 ± 12[b]
A.D. + exercise	9	243 ± 7[a]	210 ± 14

° Standard error of mean

°° 2% cholesterol + 5% cottonseed oil added to mash

°°° 750 yds. daily, 5 days per week

a $p < .01$ - controls, P.M. vs A.D. + exercise

b $p < .001$ - controls, P.M. vs A.D.

much heavier than the controls on plain mash (p < .1). Exercise
had no effect on thyroid weights, but the thyroids of the group
fed a cholesterol diet only were significantly heavier than the
exercised controls on plain mash (p < .001).

Table VI depicts the changes in the hydroxyproline concentration of collagen and elastin as well as the C/E ratio in the thoracic aortas of these birds with induced atherosclerosis. There
were no significant changes in the hydroxyproline content of collagen in any of the birds except for the atherogenic fed group
with exercise. This group was markedly lower in collagen then the
plain mash group with exercise or the group fed an atherogenic diet
only. Exercise did not have any effect on the concentration of
hydroxyproline of elastin in the thoracic aorta. Of these changes,
a more meaningful expression was the C/E ratio. Exercise had no
influence on the collagen to elastin ratio of the controls on plain
mash. However, the ratio of the atherogenic fed group with exercise
was significantly lower than that of the non-exercised birds fed a
similar diet (p < .05). It was also observed that ratio of the
exercised group fed an atherogenic regimen was markedly lower than
similarly fed exercised birds on plain mash. Further analyses were
undertaken to determine the amount of hydroxyproline and nitrogen
in the collagen extract of 100 mg of dry, lipid-free aortic tissue
(Table VII). There were no marked differences in any of the groups
with the exception of the birds on an atherogenic regimen with exercise. The amount of hydroxyproline in the group on an atherogenic
diet was significantly reduced by exercise when compared to similarly exercised birds on plain mash (p < .01). The concentration of
nitrogen in collagen extract was statistically different for only
the exercised group on a cholesterol regimen. The content of nitrogen in this group was markedly lower (p < .001) than the exercised group on plain mash. Changes in both levels of hydroxyproline
and nitrogen further confirm the significant difference observed
in the C/E ratio of the exercised birds on an atherogenic diet
when compared to the other groups.

                              DISCUSSION

Anitschow (1933) was the first to observe that feeding rabbits
a cholesterol diet for several months resulted in arterial lesions.
When these animals were returned to normal regimen, regression of
the plaques occurred, but this required an extremely long time.
It was reported by Horlick and Katz (1949) that upon cessation of
an atherogenic diet with the return of chicks to a regular non-fat
mash, hypercholesterolemia rapidly fell to normal levels.

After several weeks, regression of the lesions induced by a
cholesterol regimen was observed. Kritchevsky et al (1961, 1962) attempted, without success, to produce a regression of pre-established atheromata in animals by adding thyroid compounds and various

Table VI. Hydroxyproline Concentration of Collagen and Elastin in THORACIC Aortas of Cockerels with Induced Atherosclerosis

GROUPS	No. of Birds	Percentage hydroxyproline due to collagen	Percentage hydroxyproline due to elastin	C/E ratio
Controls, P.M.	9	$1.64 \pm 0.12°$	1.32 ± 0.07	1.31 ± 0.16
P.M. + exercise°°	9	1.71 ± 0.55	1.20 ± 0.01	1.39 ± 0.05
A.D.°°°	9	1.70 ± 0.02	1.19 ± 0.04	1.46 ± 0.14[a]
A.D. + exercise	9	1.42 ± 0.08	1.24 ± 0.07	1.15 ± 0.06[b]

° Standard error of mean

°° 750 yards daily, 5 days a week

°°° 2% cholesterol + 5% cottonseed oil added to mash

$$C/E = \frac{\text{Percent of hydroxyproline due to collagen}}{\text{Percent of hydroxyproline due to elastin}}$$

[a] $p < .05$ A.D. vs A.D. + exercise

[b] $p < .05$ A.D. + exercise vs P.M. + exercise

Table VII. Content of Hydroxyproline and Nitrogen in Collagen Extract of Dry Lipid-Free Aorta

GROUPS	No. of Birds	μM hydroxyproline in 100 mg	mM nitrogen in 100 mg
Controls, P.M.	9	12.5 ± 0.9°	.23 ± .016
P.M. + exercise°°	9	13.1 ± 0.6[a]	.27 ± .023
A.D.°°°	9	12.9 ± 1.2	.23 ± .013[b]
A.D. + exercise	9	10.7 ± 0.6	.17 ± .008

° Standard error of mean
°° 750 yds daily, 5 days a week
°°° 2% cholesterol + 5% cottonseed oil added to mash

[a] p < .01 P.M. + exercise vs A.D. + exercise

[b] p < .001 A.D. vs A.D. + exercise

fats and fatty acids in diets of animals. Thyroid administration
to chicks resulted in regression of aortic atherosclerosis was reported by Rodbard, Pick and Katz (1954). By discontinuing feeding
an atherogenic diet to rabbits, Friedman and Byers (1965) observed
the lowering of cholesterol level of the thrombo-atherosclerotic
lesion in rabbit with an implanted aortic coil. Bortz (1968) reported that aortic atherosclerosis could be reversed in cholesterol
fed rabbits if the arterial wall was exposed briefly to elevated
levels of plasma cholesterol. In this study the exercise used was
not sufficiently severe to cause a lowered plasma cholesterol in
cockerels with atherosclerosis induced by and maintained on an
atherogenic diet of plain mash mixed with 2% cholesterol and 5%
cottonseed oil by weight.

It was reported from our laboratory (1957)that the plasma
cholesterol of cockerels fed a cholesterol regimen was significantly lowered by physical activity. Later we observed that running in a treadmill resulted in a decreased level of plasma cholesterol and atherosclerosis of aortic and coronary vessels of ca-
pons fed an atherogenic diet when compared to the non-exercised
groups (1957). Similar results were obtained in chickens by Warnock et al (1957) and Orma (1957). We reported that prolonged
and intensive exercise of birds, running almost a mile daily, 5
consecutive days a week for 24 weeks resulted in a significant
lowering of the plasma cholesterol, phospholipids, triglycerides
and esterified fatty acids when compared to sedentary groups fed
a similar regimen (1966). Kobernick et al (1957) have shown that
cholesterol fed rabbits subjected to physical exercise had less
severe aortic atherosclerosis when compared to a similarly fed
sedentary group. Brown et al (1956) reported that physical activity had no consistent influence on the pathogenesis of atherosclerosis in rabbits receiving low or high cholesterol diets.
Recent studies by Link and his associates (1972) indicate that
feeding pigs an atherogenic diet increased the plasma lipids.
No significant sex differences in plasma cholesterol, total lipids,
triglycerides and plasma fibrinogen was observed. There were marked differences however, in the degree of atherosclerosis between
the exercised and non-exercised pigs. The exercised animals ate
more, gained less weight, had less atherosclerosis and less total
body fat than the non-exercised pigs. It was observed that the
weight of the heart was heavier in the exercised group as compared
to the non-exercised. Studies from our laboratory (1969) have
shown that artificial pacing of the hearts in cockerels at almost
twice the normal heart rate resulted in a marked decrease in plasma
cholesterol levels as well as reducing the severity of aortic atherosclerosis. The heart and adrenal weights were much heavier than
the non-paced groups on plain mash or on an atherogenic regimen.
The exercise used was not stressful as is indicated by the slight
increase in the adrenal weights of the birds on plain mash or on

a cholesterol diet. Studies from our laboratory show that if
chickens were severely stressed on a treadmill, there would be
a significant enlargement of the adrenal glands (1966). According to Conner and Shaffner (1954) this increase was due to hyper-
trophy and hyperplasia of both cortical and medullary tissue.
Increasing the cockerel heart rate from approximately 240 beats
per minute to 420 or 480 BPM by a pacemaker resulted in an increase in adrenal weights (1969, 1971). Although the plasma cholesterol level of the exercised group fed an atherogenic diet was
not significantly different from the non-exercised birds, physical
activity reduced the severity of aortic and coronary atherosclerosis of birds which had been induced by and maintained on a high
cholesterol regimen. Results from this study indicate that the
hydroxyproline concentration of collagen was not influenced by
exercise and that the only decrease observed was in the atherogenic fed group with exercise. Our values are lower than those
reported by Cembrano and his colleagues (1960) and Nichols et al
(1971). The former also reported sex differences and hormonal
effects on the concentration of collagen and elastin in aortas
of five to six month old Leghorn chickens. Cockerels were either
castrated or 25 mg estradiol pellets were implanted in the sub-
cutaneous tissue of the neck. Pullets were treated with testosterone. A month or two later these birds were sacrificed and
analyzed for the hydroxyproline content of collagen and elastin.
It was observed that both these concentrations were higher in
cockerels than in pullets. They suggested this difference was possibly due to testosterone, since it was noted that cockerels following castration, had collagen and elastin levels in the aortas
similar to those observed in pullets. When male hormone was ad-
ministered to pullets, the collagen and elastin concentration was
increased to almost the same level as that of cockerels.

When cockerels were treated with estradiol the amount of collagen and elastin in the aorta was significantly reduced. In the
latter study young birds of 62 days of age were used for given
intervals 0.5, 1.5, 3 or 5 months. They reported that the level
of hydroxyproline in the abdominal portion of the controls, diethyl-
stilbesterol treated and groups fed 0.5% cholesterol showed an increase with time, and that it was significantly higher than the concentration found in the thoracic area. Also the abdominal portion
of the aorta had more collagen than the thoracic while the opposite
was true for elastin. Our studies showed that physical activity
did not have a significant influence on the hydroxyproline level
of elastin. The concentration of hydroxyproline of elastin for our
controls on plain mash was similar to that reported by Cembrano et
al (1960) and Nichols et al (1971). The latter observed that there
were no significant differences in the elastin contents of chicken
aorta of controls, DES treated or those fed 0.5% cholesterol. The
only marked decrease in elastin was observed in the cholesterol

fed group at the end of one and a half months. These investigators also reported that the collagen to elastin ratio of the
thoracic aorta was significantly higher in this group when compared to the controls. Our study showed that exercise had no effect
on the collagen to elastin ratio of cockerels on plain mash, but
the cholesterol fed group which was exercised had a significantly
lower C/E ratio as compared to a similarly fed non-exercised group.
It has been suggested by Kramsch and Hollander (1973) that the
mechanism involved in the deposition of lipids in arterial elastin
may be due to an interaction of the elastin protein to LDL or VLDL.
Since a decrease in the C/E ratio also indicates a lower concentration of collagen and elastin, we can only speculate that this may
explain the phenomena observed in our study whereby there was a
reversal in the severity of aortic atherosclerosis of exercise
cockerels with induced atherosclerosis when compared to a similarly fed sedentary group even though the plasma cholesterol of these
two groups was not significantly different. Our results seem to
confirm the hypothesis of Kramsch and Hollander (1971) that the
focal lipid deposition observed in early atherosclerotic lesions
is due to lipid accumulations in altered elastin protein of localized areas in the intima. The authors postulated that elastin of
intimal elastin membrane may have an important role in the pathogenesis of atherosclerotic process. Wolinsky (1972) observed that
in short-term hypertension there was a disproportionate elevation
in noncollagenous alkali-soluble proteins which he attributed to
be due to the vascular smooth muscle, whereas in long-term hypertension no further increase in these proteins was noticed although
there were increases in mural accumulations of collagen and elastin.
Studies by Mack et al (1970) demonstrated that in rabbits the total
amount of mature collagen in the aorta was decreased from 25% in
the controls to 21% in animals with atherosclerosis. They also reported no appreciable changes were observed in the total ratio of
elastin extracted from old cows' aortas when compared to young.

REFERENCES

1. Anitschkow, N.
   Experimental Atherosclerosis in Animals.
   In Artiosclerosis: Review of Problem, edited by E.V. Cowdry,
   Macmillan, New York, pp. 271-322, 1933.
2. Bortz, W.M.
   Reversibility of Atherosclerosis in Cholesterol-Fed Rabbits.
   Circulation Res. XXII: 135, 1968.
3. Brown, C.E., Huang, T.C., Bortz, E.L. and McCay, C.:
   Observations on Blood Vessels and Exercise.
   J. Geront. 11: 292, 1956.
4. Burton, A.C.:
   Relation of Structure to Function of the Tissues of
   Blood Vessels.
   Physiol. Rev. 34: 619, 1954.

5. Cembrano, J., Lillo, M., Val, J. and Mardones, J.:
   Influence of Sex Difference and Hormones on Elastin and
   Collagen in the Aorta of Chickens·
   Circulation Res. VIII: 527, 1960·
6. Conner, M. H. and Shaffner, C.S.: Effect of Altered
   Thyroidal and Gonadal Activity on Size of Endocrine
   Glands and Resistance to Stress in the Chick·
   Endocrinology 55: 45, 1954.
7. Fischer, G.M.: In Vivo Effects of Estradiol on Collagen
   and Elastin in Rat Aorta.
   Endocrinology 91: 1227, 1972.
8. Fischer, G.M. and Llaurado, J.G.: Collagen and Elastin
   Content in Canine Arteries Selected from Functionally
   Different Vascular Beds.
   Circulation Res. 19: 394, 1966.
9. Fischer, G.M. and Llaurado, J.G.:
   Connective Tissue Composition of Human Coronary Artery
   and its Relationship to Divalent Cation Content.
   Angiology 22: 31, 1971.
10. Friedman, M. and Byers, S.O.: Immunity of the Mature
    Thromboatherosclerotic Plaque to Hypercholesterolemia.
    Brit. J. Exptl. Pathol. 46: 539, 1965.
11. Histologic Staining Methods of Armed Forces
    Institute of Pathology, edited by L. Luna, McGraw Hill,
    New York, p. 140, 1968
12. Horlick, L. and Katz, L.N.: Retrogression of Atherosclerotic
    Lesions on Cessation of Cholesterol Feeding in the Chick.
    J. Lab. & Clin. Med. 34: 1427, 1949.
13. Houck, J.C. and Jacob, R.A.: Effect of Age Upon Collagen
    and Hexosamine Content of Rat Skin.
    Proc. Soc. Exptl. Biol. Med. 97: 604, 1954.
14. Katz, L.N. and Stamler, J.: Experimental Atherosclerosis,
    C.C. Thomas, Springfield, Illinois, p. 136, 1953.
15. Kobernick, S.D., Niwayama, G. and Zuchlewski, A.C.:
    Effect of Physical Activity on Cholesterol
    Atherosclerosis in Rabbits.
    Proc. Soc. Exper. Biol. Med. 96: 623, 1953.
16. Kramsch, D.M., Franzblau, C. and Hollander, W.:
    The Protein and Lipid Composition of Arterial Elastin and
    its Relationship to Lipid Accumulation in the Atherosclerotic
    Plaque.
    J. Clin. Invest. 50: 1666, 1971.
17. Kramsch, D.M. and Hollander, W.:
    The Interaction of Serum and Arterial Lipoproteins with
    Elastin of the Arterial Intima and its Role in the Lipid
    Accumulation in Atherosclerotic Plaques.
    J. Clin. Invest. 52: 236, 1973.

18. Kritchevsky, D., Moynihan, J.L., Langan, J., Tepper, S.A. and Sacks, M.L.: Effects of D- and L- Thyroxine and D- and L- 3, 5, 3' - triiodo - Thyronine in Development and Regression of Experimental Atherosclerosis in Rabbits. J. Atherosclerosis Res. 1: 211, 1961.
19. Kritchevsky, D. and Tepper, S.A.: Cholesterol Vehicle in Experimental Atherosclerosis. V. Influence of Fats and Fatty Acids on Pre-Established Atheromata. J. Atherosclerosis Res. 2: 471, 1962.
20. Link, R.P., Pedersoli, W.M. and Satanie, A.H.: Effect of Exercise on Development of Atherosclerosis in Swine. Atherosclerosis 15: 107, 1972.
21. Mack, G., Ebel, A., Kemf, E.E., Pantesco, V., Fontaine, J.L. and Fontaine, R.: Aortic Aging and its Connection with Arteriosclerosis. Experimental Research. J. Thor. Cardiovasc. Surg. 11: 292, 1970.
22. Malinow, M.R. and Perley, A.: The Effect of Physical Exercise on Cholesterol Degradation in Man. J. Atheroscler. Res. 10: 107, 1969.
23. Malinow, M.R., McLaughlin, P.A. and Perley, A.: The Effect of Muscular Contraction on Cholesterol Oxidation. J. Appl. Physiol. 25: 733, 1968.
24. Malinow, M.R., McLaughlin, P.A. and Perley, A.: Treadmill Activity Accelerates Cholesterol Oxidation in Rats. Science 160: 1239, 1968.
25. Mann, G.V., Teal, K., Hayes, O., McNally, A. and Bruno, W.: Exercise in the Disposition of Dietary Calories. New Engl. J. Med. 253: 349, 1955.
26. Newman, R.E. and Logan, M.A.: The Determination of Collagen and Elastin in Tissues. J. Biol. Chem. 186: 549, 1950.
27. Nichols, C.W. Jr., Gan, J.C., Murthy, P.V.N. and Chaikoff, I.L.: Mucosubstances in the Chicken Aorta. Atherosclerosis 14: 39, 1971.
28. Orma, E.J.: Effect of Physical Activity on Atherogenesis: An Experimental Study in Cockerels. Acta. Physiol. Scand. 41: suppl. 142: 1, 1957.
29. Rodbard, S., Pick, R. and Katz, L.N.: Rate of Regression of Hypercholesterolemia and Atherosclerosis in Chicks. Effects of Diet, Pancreatectomy, Estrogens and Thyroid. Circulation 10: 547, 1954.
30. Warnock, N.H., Clarkson, T.B. and Stevenson, R.: Effect of Exercise on Blood Coagulation Time and Atherosclerosis in Cholesterol-fed Cockerels. Circulation Res. 5: 478, 1957.
31. Wolinsky, H.: Long-term Effects of Hypertension on the Rat Aortic Wall and their Relation to Current Aging Changes: Morphological and Chemical Studies. Circulation Res. XXX: 301, 1972.

32. Wong, H.Y.C., Johnson, F.B. and Wong, A.K.:
    The Effects of Exercise and Androgen on
    Cholesterol-fed Capons.
    Circulation 16: 501, 1957.
33. Wong, H.Y.C., Loh, S.J., Bonucelli, H.A. and Johnson, F.B.:
    Effects of Increasing Heart Rate on Plasma Cholesterol
    and Atherosclerosis of Cholesterol-fed Cockerels.
    Fed. Proc. 28: No. 2, 1424, 1969.
34. Wong, H.Y.C., Mendez, H.C. and Johnson, F.B.:
    The Effect of Prolonged and Intensive Exercise on Blood
    Lipids and Atherosclerosis of Cholesterol-fed Cockerels.
    Fed. Proc. 25: 759, 1966.
35. Wong, H.Y.C., Mendez, H.C., Walters, C.S. and Orvis, H.H.:
    A Revised Method for Determination of Total Plasma
    Cholesterol in Blood.
    Life Sci. 4: 431, 1965.
36. Wong, H.Y.C., Simmons, R., Kim, J., Liu, D. and
    Hawthorne, E.W.: Hypocholesterolizing Effect of
    Exercise on Cholesterol-fed Cockerels.
    Fed. Proc. 16: 138, 1957.
37. Wong, H.Y.C., Tchuisse, M.L., Baird, G., Cock, A. and
    Loh, S.J.: Exercise or Pacing Effects on Plasma Cholesterol,
    Atherosclerosis, Heart and Adrenal Weights of Cockerels.
    Fed. Proc. 30: No. 2, 2518, 1971.

Supported by National Institutes of Health, Grant #RR08016.

DIET AND HUMAN ATHEROSCLEROSIS - CARBOHYDRATES

I. MACDONALD

Department of Physiology

Guy's Hospital Medical School, London SE1 9RT

Only recently have dietary carbohydrates been considered to play a harmful part in health. For thousands of years peoples have been consuming large quantities of carbohydrate, mainly because they are the basis of cheap food and because they satisfy hunger, and it was the dentists that were the first to point out that dietary carbohydrates could produce pathological lesions. Then in 1961 (1) it was reported that the level of triglyceride in the fasting serum seemed to be directly related to the amount of carbohydrate eaten.

If the preseumption is made that the level of lipids in the fasting serum bears some relationship to the extent of atherosclerosis and its complications (5) then it is logical to study the effects that dietary carbohydrates have on the level of various lipid fractions in the serum. If the incidence of carbohydrate-induced-hyperlipidaemia in males aged 25-79 years is indeed 10-13% as has been reported (37, 40) then the role of diatary carbohydrates in the genesis of atherosclerosis may be far from negligible.

As triglyceride is the principal lipid fraction in the serum influenced by dietary carbohydrate, then it is necessary to study the effects on serum triglyceride of variations such as the amount and type of dietary carbohydrate, the chronological relationship to the time of carbohydrate consumption, the influence of other dietary factors accompanying the carbohydrate and the "sensitivity" of the consumer.

CHRONOLOGICAL RELATIONSHIP BETWEEN DIETARY
CARBOHYDRATE AND SERUM TRIGLYCERIDE LEVELS

When considering this aspect of the dietary carbohydrate/
lipid/atherosclerosis relationship there appears to be conflict.
When glucose from starch and starch derivatives in the diet is
absorbed the serum triglyceride concentration falls during the
subsequent few hours (10). Similarly the lipaemia following a
meal containing 60 g of fat can be abolished by adding 100-250 g
of glucose to the meal (2). This acute lowering of serum triglyceride level by carbohydrate also occurs if glucose is given
intravenously (13) thus eliminating an absorption factor.

The explanation for this immediate lowering of serum triglyceride by glucose probably lies in the fact that the insulin,
released by glucose, stimulates lipo-protein lipase activity (15).
Support for this view comes from the finding that insulin given
to hypertriglyceridaemic patients causes a fall in serum triglyceride (35) and that the administration of fructose – which is not an
effective stimulus to insulin release – causes less marked reduction in serum triglyceride levels (8, 28).

Thus it seems that, if a raised serum triglyceride level is
undesirable, then one immediate method of reducing this level is
to give an insulin stimulating carbohydrate such as glucose.
Unfortunately, the carbohydrate/lipid relationship is not so simple
as this because as has been reported (1) a diet high in carbohydrate raises the fasting serum triglyceride level.

It would perhaps be wise to digress for a moment and to discuss this conflicting role of dietary carbohydrates in triglyceride metabolism, and hence possible atherosclerosis. It is not
known whether it is the overall mean level of serum triglyceride
which is a cause of atherosclerosis, or whether in the aetiology
of atherosclerosis the important triglycerides are those we consume
(exogenous) or those we make (endogenous). If it is overall serum
triglyceride level that is important then frequent ingestion of
small quantities of glucose or its polymers would seem advisable.
If in some way the endogenous triglycerides are responsible for
atherosclerosis then reduced intake of dietary carbohydrate by those
who have a propensity to convert carbohydrate to triglyceride
would be advisable. As, at this moment, it is not known which if
either, view is correct, then it would, perhaps be wise to consider
in more detail the role of dietary carbohydrates in endogenous triglyceride metabolism.

When most normal men increase the proportion of carbohydrate
in their diet the level of the triglyceride in their fasting serum
increases at first before gradually returning to normal (3). In
those whose fasting serum triglyceride level is raised an increase
in the proportion of dietary carbohydrate causes a more marked rise
which will not, if the increased carbohydrate intake persists, re-

turn to normal values (7). This group of patients are the so-called "carbohydrate-induced" hyperlipoproteinaemias or Fredrickson's type IV. As this carbohydrate-induced hypertriglyceridaemia is associated with vascular disease then it is obviously necessary to advise such a person to reduce the intake of carbohydrate.

FRUCTOSE AND ATHEROSCLEROSIS

There is evidence that in men, at least in the short term, the carbohydrate sucrose causes a more marked rise in the fasting serum triglyceride level than does glucose or its polymers (14, 17, 22) whereas the substitution of glucose for starch in the diet of two hyperglyceridaemic patients did not result in any deterioration of triglyceride level (33). In one study in which sucrose in the diet was replaced by glucose syrup in men whose level of triglyceride was raised, the replacement of sucrose was accompanied by a fall in fasting triglyceride levels (34).

The feature of sucrose that distinguishes it from other common dietary carbohydrates is that it contains fructose, and in experiments in animals (11, 30) and man (18) it has been reported that fructose raises the level of fasting serum triglyceride more than does glucose. It is unlikely that fructose forms more triglyceride overall than does glucose (29) because of the greater lipogenesis, under the influence of insulin, of glucose in adipose tissue. However, fructose (or sucrose) does seem to result in increased hepatic lipogenesis and raised endogenous triglyceride levels in the serum (41). Metabolic studies in the rat (24) and in the monkey (25) as well as in healthy men and men who have recovered from a myocardial infarct (20) would support the hypothesis that more fructose than glucose is converted to serum triglyceride.

In this context it is of interest to note that in patients with peripheral vascular disease given a load of sucrose, the subsequent level of serum fructose is considerably higher than in a comparable group with no evidence of vascular disease(27). Furthermore the level of serum fructose is higher after a dose of sucrose than after a comparable dose of its constituent monosaccharides glucose and fructose (26).

It would seem from the foregoing that fructose as such or in sucrose can be undesirable in terms of triglyceridaemia, but it should perhaps be remembered that fructose can be converted by the liver to glucose and that perhaps only when large quantities are consumed does this conversion mechanism become overwhelmed and allow fructose to be matabolised as such. Also, as will be seen later, there are other factors which modify the metabolic response to fructose.

SOME FACTORS THAT MODIFY THE LIPID RESPONSE
TO DIETARY CARBOHYDRATE

1. Type of fat accompanying the carbohydrate - There is a
tendency in nutritional/metabolic studies to consider the component of the diet under investigation in isolation. We do not eat
single components but a mixture of various types of food, and it
is therefore important to consider whether an effect found when
one food is given in isolation, and probably in excess, is present
when that food is eaten in combination with other foods.

The effect that dietary fats have on dietary carbohydrate metabolism is just such an example. Sucrose or fructose in large enough
quantities raise the level of endogenous triglycerides in the serum
- at least in the short-term. When sucrose or fructose are given
with a saturated fath such as cream, the response of the endogenous
triglyceride level is unaffected, but when the saturated fat is replaced by a polyunsaturated fat such as sunflower seed oil, the rise
in fasting serum triglycerides in response to sucrose or fructose
does not occur. In fact the reverse takes place and the triglyceride level falls (19, 31, 21).

Furthermore, the physiological rise in serum triglycerides
(exogenous) after a meal containing fat is reduced by adding carbohydrate and especially glucose or its polymers to the meal (2).
This effect may not be seen when fructose or glycerol accompany
the dietary fat (32).

2. Sex of the consumer - It is an interesting fact that the
incidence of atherosclerosis and its consequences is much lower
in pre-menopausal women than in men of a comparable age group (38,
39). It is also an interesting observation that the increased level of triglyceride in the fasting serum found when there is an increase in sucrose or fructose in the diet of young men does not occur when similar diets are given to young women (4, 16). There is
also some experimental evidence to suggest that the oral contraceptive together with dietary sucrose raises the level of fasting
serum triglyceride to a greater extent than either alone (38).

3. Other modifying factors - The frequency of consuming large
quantities of sucrose (23) and the nitrogen source accompanying
sucrose (6) have been shown to alter the fasting serum triglyceride response to sucrose. There are doubtless many other interrelationships important and as yet unknown.

DIETARY CARBOHYDRATES AND SERUM CHOLESTEROL

Diets high in carbohydrate cause a fall in serum cholesterol (9, 36) and the fall is less when sucrose is the principal carbohydrate (12). The effect that dietary carbohydrate has on serum cholesterol is very likely to be secondary to such causes as the replacement of saturated fat by carbohydrate, or the rise in endogenous serum triglyceride cuased by carbohydrate means a rise in pre-beta lipoprotein and this lipoprotein contains a small amount of cholesterol.

CONCLUSIONS

There is not sufficient evidence at the moment to be dogmatic about the role of dietary carbohydrates in atherosclerosis. What therefore is the practising physician to do when faced with giving dietary advice in either the prevention or treatment of atherosclerosis?

1. Learn whether the patient is "carbohydrate-sensitive". This can be done by determining the level of serum triglyceride after a 12-14 hour fast, and if possible get confirmation that any increase is in the pre-beta lipoprotein (VLDL).

2. If the patient is "carbohydrate-sensitive" reduce his intake of carbohydrate, paying particular attention to sucrose and honey, as these are major sources of fructose.

3. Persuade the patient to eat more polyunsaturated fat and less animal fat, as the polyunsaturated fat will offset the effect of dietary carbohydrate on fasting serum triglyceride levels.

4. If the "carbohydrate-sensitive" patient is taking an oral contraceptive it is possible that withdrawal of this type of contraceptive will reduce the extent of the "carbohydrate-sensitivity".

5. Weight reduction will frequently make the patient no longer "carbohydrate-sensitive".

REFERENCES

1. Ahrens, E.H., Hirsch, S., Oettle, K., Farquhar, J.W. and Stein, Y.: Carbohydrate-induced and fat-induced lipemia Trans. Ass. Amer. Physicians 74: 134-146, 1961.
2. Albrink, M.J., Fitzgerald, J.R. and Man, E.B.: Reduction of alimentary lipemia by glucose Metabolism 7: 162-171, 1958.
3. Antonis, A. and Bersohn, I.: The influence of diet on serum triglycerides in South African White and Bantu prisoners Lancet i: 3-9, 1961.

4. Beveridge, J.M.R., Jagannathan, S.N. and Connell, W.F.:
   The effect of the type and amount of dietary fat on the
   level of plasma triglycerides in human subjects in the
   postabsorptive state.
   Canad. J. Biochem. 42: 999–1003, 1964.
5. Carlson, L.A. and Böttiger, L.E.: Ischaemic heart disease
   in relation to fasting values of plasma triglycerides and
   cholesterol
   Lancet i: 865–868, 1972.
6. Coles, B.L. and MacDonald, I.: The influence of dietary protein
   on dietary carbohydrate: lipid interrelationships
   Nutr. Metab. 14: 238–244, 1972.
7. Farquhar, J.W., Frank, A., Gross, R.C. and Reaven, G.M.:
   Glucose, insulin and triglyceride responses to high and
   low carbohydrate diets. J. Clin. Invest. 45: 1648–1656, 1966.
8. Grodsky, G.M., Batts, A.A., Bennett, L.L., Vcella, C.,
   McWilliams, N.B. and Smith, D.: Effects of carbohydrates
   on secretion of insulin from isolated rat pancreas
   Amer. J. Physiol. 205: 638–644, 1963.
9. Hatch, F.T., Abell, L.L. and Kendall, F.E.: Effects of
   restriction of dietary fat and cholesterol upon serum
   lipids and lipoproteins in patients with hypertension
   Amer. J. Med. 19: 48–60, 1955.
10. Havel, R.J.: Early effects of fasting and of carbohydrate
    ingestion on lipids and lipoproteins of serum in man
    J. Clin. Invest. 36: 855–859, 1957.
11. Hill, P.: Effect of fructose on rat lipids
    Lipids 5: 621–627, 1969.
12. Hodges, R.E. and Krehl, W.A.: The role of carbohydrate
    in lipid metabolism
    Amer. J. Clin. Nutr. 17: 334–346, 1965.
13. Jourdan, M.H.: The effect of a sucrose-enriched diet on the
    metabolism of intravenously administered fructose in baboons
    Nutr. Metab. 14: 28–37, 1972.
14. Kaufmann, N.A., Poznanski, R., Blondheim, S.A. and Stein, Y.:
    Changes in serum lipid levels of hyperlipemic patients following
    the feeding of starch, sucrose and glucose
    Amer. J. Clin. Nutr. 18: 261–269, 1966.
15. Kessler, J.I.: Effect of insulin on the release of plasma
    lipolytic activity and clearing of emulsified fat intra-
    venously administered to pancreatectomised and alloxanised
    dogs
    J. Lab. Clin. Med. 60: 747–755, 1962.
16. Klugh, C.A. and Irwin, M.I.: Serum levels of young women as
    related to source of dietary carbohydrate
    Fed. Proc. 25: 672, 1966.
17. Kuo, P.T. and Bassett, D.R.: Dietary sugar in the production
    of hyperglyceridemia
    Ann. Intern. Med. 62: 1199–1212, 1965.

18. MacDonald, I.: Influence of fructose and glucose on serum lipid levels in men and pre- and post-menopausal women. Amer. J. Clin. Nutr. 18: 369-372, 1966.

19. MacDonald, I.: Interrelationship between the influence of dietary carbohydrates and fats on fasting serum lipids. Amer. J. Clin. Nutr. 20: 345-351, 1967.

20. MacDonald, I.: Ingested glucose and fructose in serum lipids in healthy men and after myocardial infarction. Amer. J. Clin. Nutr. 21: 1366-1373, 1968.

21. MacDonald, I.: Relationship between dietary carbohydrates and fats in their influence on serum lipid levels. Clin. Sci. 43: 265-274, 1972.

22. MacDonald, I. and Braithwaite, D.M.: The influence of dietary carbohydrates on the lipid pattern in serum and in adipose tissue. Clin. Sci. 27: 23-30, 1964.

23. MacDonald, I., Coles, B.L., Brice, J. and Jourdan, M.H.: The influence of frequency of sucrose intake on serum lipid, and carbohydrate levels. Brit. J. Nutr. 24: 413-423, 1970

24. MacDonald, I. and Roberts, J.B.: The incorporation of various ^{14}C dietary carbohydrates into serum and liver lipids. Metabolism 14: 991-999, 1965.

25. MacDonald, I. and Roberts, J.B.: The serum lipid response of baboons to various carbohydrate meals. Metabolism 16: 572-579, 1967.

26. MacDonald, I. and Turner, L.J.: Serum fructose levels after sucrose or its constituent monosaccharides. Lancet i: 841-843, 1968.

27. MacDonald, I. and Turner, L.J.: Serum glucose and fructose levels after sucrose meals in atherosclerosis. Nutr. Metab. 13: 168-171, 1971.

28. Mann, J.I., Truswell, A.S. and Pimstone, B.L.: The different effects of oral sucrose and glucose on alimentary lipemia. Clin. Sci. 41: 123-129, 1971.

29. Maruhama, Y. and MacDonald, I.: Some changes in the triglyceride metabolism of rats on high fructose or glucose diets. Metabolism 21: 835-842, 1972.

30. Mukherjee, S., Baso, M. and Trivedi, K.: Effect of low dietary levels of glucose, fructose and sucrose on rat lipid metabolism. J. Atheroscler. Res. 10: 261-272, 1969.

31. Nestel, P.J., Carroll, K.F. and Havenstein, N.: Plasma triglyceride response to carbohydrates, fats and calorie intake. Metabolism 19: 1-18, 1970

32. Nikkila, E.A. and Pelkonen, R.: Enhancement of alimentary hyperglyceridemia by fructose and glycerol in man. Proc. Soc. Exp. Biol. Med. 123: 91-94, 1966.

33. Porte, D., Bierman, E.L. and Bagdade, J.D.: Substitution
    of dietary starch for dextrose in hyperlipemic subjects.
    Proc. Soc. Exp. Biol. Med. 123: 814-816.
34. Roberts, A.M.: Effects of a sucrose-free diet on the serum-
    lipid levels of men in Antarctica.
    Lancet i: 1201-1204, 1973.
35. Schlierf, G. and Kinsell, R.: Effect of insulin in hyper-
    triglyceridemia.
    Proc. Soc.Exp. Biol. Med. 120: 272-274, 1965.
36. Starke, H.: Effect of the rice diet on the serum cholesterol
    fractions of one hundred and fifty four patients with hyper-
    tensive vascular disease.
    Amer. J. Med. 9: 494-499, 1950.
37. Stone, M.C. and Dick, T.B.S.: Prevalence of hyperlipo-
    proteinemias in a random sample of men and in patients
    with ischaemic heart disease.
    Brit. Heart J. 35: 954-961, 1973.
38. Stovein, V. and MacDonald, I.: Some effects of diet with
    oral contraceptives on carbohydrate: lipid metabolism in
    the baboon. Proc. Nutr. Soc. 32:34A.
39. Taylor, R.D., Corcoran, A.C. and Page, I.H.: Menopausal
    hypertension. Critical study.
    Amer. J. Med. Sci. 213: 475-476, 1947.
40. Wood, P.D.S., Stern, M.P., Silvers, A., Reaven, G.M.
    and Groenen, J.: Prevalence of plasma lipoprotein
    abnormalities in a free-living population of the Central
    Valley, California.
    Circulation 45: 114-126, 1972.
41. Zakim, D.: Influence of fructose on hepatic synthesis of
    lipids.
    Progress in Biochem. Pharm. Vol. 8. Karger, Basel, 1974.

THE EFFECTS OF FEEDING VARIOUS DIETARY FATS ON THE DEVELOPMENT AND REGRESSION OF HYPERCHOLESTEROLEMIA AND ATHEROSCLEROSIS

R.W. WISSLER AND D. VESSELINOVITCH

The Department of Pathology and Specialized Center of

Research in Atherosclerosis at the University of Chicago

The factors responsible for the development of atherosclerosis and the dietary lipids influencing it can only be studied under well controlled conditions in the experimental animal (1). Among the many experimental models of this disease process that have been investigated, the progressive atheromatous arterial lesions produced in the Rhesus monkey utilizing the nutritional approaches pioneered by Taylor et al (2,3,4) offer a number of advantages. The Rhesus monkey atheormatous lesions tend to resemble the human disease process much more closely in morphologic characteristics, distribution and complications than those frequently studied in the rabbit, rat, fowl and dog. The large number of additional advantages and the relatively few disadvantages of using the Rhesus monkey model of atherosclerosis produced by dietary means have been reviewed recently (5) and will not be repeated here. Suffice it to say that most of the disadvantages of this experimental model can be overcome by diligent work.

The model lesions produced by dietary means in swine offer some of the same advantages (6). However, the swine model seems to have the disadvantages of not readily progressing to the advanced stage of atherosclerosis that is usually responsible for the clinical effects of coronary stenosis or occlusion and the other ischemic clinical effects. Thus far these clinical complications have only been produced in swine by utilizing "catheter injury" or "high dosage x-ray" exposure of the heart (8) to augment the dietarily induced

Supported in part by grants HE 2174, HL 6894 and HL 15062 from the National Heart and Lung Institute of the National Institutes of Health, United States Public Health Service.

65

lesions - and even then the distribution of the advanced lesions
may be quite different from those usually developing in man. Furthermore, there is some evidence that adult swine often develop
severe, widespread, spontaneous, small artery smooth muscle proli-
ferative lesions in the myocardium that are rare in man (9). In
any event it appears to be of value when studying dietary factors
to use a model that is not complicated by arterial injury or spontaneous arterial intimal or medial cell proliferation.

Earlier work in our laboratory has revealed that advanced aortic and coronary artery atherosclerosis can be produced in the Rhesus monkey in 9 months utilizing a 50:50 mixture of coconut oil and
butter fat enriching a monkey "stock" ration which also has been
altered by adding cholesterol (10). The apparent accelerated atherogenic effect of coconut oil may be related to its stimulation of
arterial cell proliferation (11). The severe atherogenicity of
this food fat has also been demonstrated by others (12,13). The
fully developed lesions produced by this dietary mixture of high
concentrations of coconut oil, butter fat and cholesterol have most
of the characteristics of those seen in advanced atherosclerosis in
man. They often display in a single lesion marked intimal cell proliferation, a large grumous lipid rich necrotic center, cholesterol
crystals, calcification at the base of the lesion, a variable amount
of new collagen and elastin in the "fibrous cap" that forms over the
necrotic area, and substantial involvement and thinning of the media under the lesion (10). Furthermore, the coronary artery lesions
are focal plaques which are largely confined to the proximal part
of each of the main coronary arteries and often cause severe narrowing of the coronary artery lumens. Only in the extremely advanced
form of the disease does the involvement of the main coronary arteries become more diffuse.

We have now studied 42 Rhesus monkeys fed this severely atherogenic ration for approximately 9 months. Fig. 1 indicates that most
of these animals had substantial aortic atherosclerosis and that in
general the extent of the disease was closely related to the level
of serum cholesterol that the animal sustained during the dietary
period.

During the course of these studies we also investigated the
comparative atherogenic effects of corn oil, butter oil and peanut
oil. Each of these food fats was fed in equal quantities to 6 Rhesus monkeys in diets that were otherwise comparable in all other
respects. In spite of relatively less elevation in blood lipids
in the monkeys fed the peanut oil ration (as compared to those fed
the butter oil diet) the animals receiving the peanut oil consistently had the most severe lesions in their aortas (14). Furthermore,
the atheromatous plaques produced by peanut oil were much thicker
and much richer in collagen than in those lesions produced by either
of the other 2 fats.

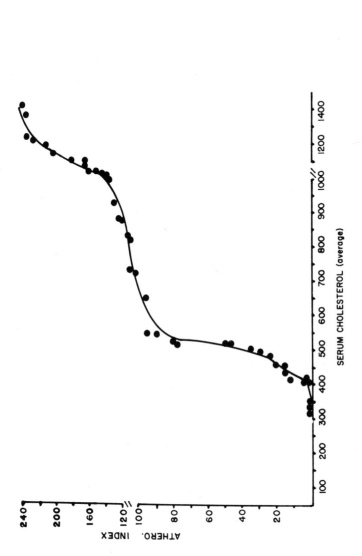

Fig. 1. A demonstration of the direct correlation between sustained serum cholesterol level and the extent and severity of aortic atherosclerosis developing in 9 months in 42 male Rhesus monkeys fed coconut oil-butter fat enriched primate rations with 2% cholesterol added. Note the remarkable upswing of lesions above 400 mg% and the relative plateau between 500 and 1000 mg%.

More recently we have extended these studies to the coronary
arteries of these same animals with similar results (15). A full
report of this work, including a study of the coronary arteries of
these animals is now in press (16). We have also been assisting
Dr. David Kritchevsky at the Wistar Institute to see if we can
learn more about the pathogenesis of the severe atherosclerosis
following the feeding of the peanut oil ration (17,18). These studies suggest that a part of the unexpected atherogenicity of peanut
oil may be related to its content of arachidic and behenic acids
(17). On the other hand some of the severe atherogenicity may be
related to the arrangement of the fatty acids in the triglycerides
of the peanut oil (18).

It must be emphasized that dietary cholesterol and some degree
of hypercholemia are necessary to demonstrate this special atherogenicity of peanut oil. The fact that very severe atherosclerosis
results from feeding cholesterol along with peanut oil even when
the serum cholesterol concentration is relatively low does not really conflict with the usual excellent correlation between the habitual serum cholesterol level and the severity of atherosclerosis
in this species. It simply indicates that other dietary factors
such as fatty acid composition of the food fat may also have great
effects on arterial cell proliferation and collagen formation.

These studies and those of others indicate that peanut oil is
more atherogenic than one would expect from its polyunsaturated
fatty acid content when it is fed as the sole source of fat in a
cholesterol-containing ration to rats (19,20), Rhesus monkeys (21),
swine (22) and rabbits (23). In general these peanut oil lesions
are characterized by severe arterial intimal cell proliferation and
abundant collagen formation with relatively little lipid deposition
- the latter being usually located deep in the lesion.

Coconut oil is also a very atherogenic lipid when fed in a
cholesterol containing ration to the Cebus monkey (11), the rat
(24) or to the dog and the rabbit (12,25,26) and the Rhesus monkey
(10). These arterial lesions also show unusually severe arterial
intimal proliferation but they frequently include abundant lipid
deposition and relatively little collagen deposition. These studies
indicate that some vegetable oils can be very atherogenic when fed
in large quantities with high intakes of cholesterol. Additional
work is necessary to ascertain whether these effects in experimental
animals have implications for the development of atherosclerosis in
man. It must be admitted that use of very large amounts of dietary
cholesterol along with large quantities of a single food fat fed as
almost the sole source of lipid in the diet over a long period
time is quite different from the usual nutritional pattern in man
even when the cholesterol and fat are combined with a mixed monkey
ration that is formulated to be a completely nutritious diet for
primates.

We have also used the Rhesus monkey to study the effects of table-prepared human diets on the development of atherosclerosis (27,28). The main purpose of these experiments was to compare the effects of a prototype of an "average" American diet with a "prudent" American diet designed to include fewer calories, less fat, especially reduced amounts of saturated food fats and less dietary cholesterol. The average American ration included 25 ingredients in the proportions consumed by American as judged by food consumption tables. The prudent ration contained 17 different ingredients. In both instances the food substances were prepared as if they were to be served to people and then they were mixed together to form a paste-like food which was fed in one large portion each day which the monkeys relished. Among those foods omitted in the prudent ration were eggs, beef fat, pork fat, liver, cheese, pound cake, saturated margarine, butter and bacon. Among the ingredients common to both diets but which were reduced substantially in the prudent ration were roast beef, roast pork and sugar.

The analyses of these rations and the basic food components consumed are shown in Table I. A complete listing of the food stuffs used and their amounts has been published recently (29) and a much more complete report on these studies is being prepared.

In 3 consecutive 2 year experiments with these rations there was a consistent contrast in the serum cholesterol levels between the 2 groups with almost all of the monkeys fed the average American diet above 300 mg% while the monkeys fed the prudent American diet maintained much lower serum cholesterol levels, usually below 250 mg%. There was also a consistent difference in the extent and severity of the atherosclerotic lesions developing in the aortas and coronary arteries of the two groups.

The results showed that aortic lesions (plaques) in animals on the average American diet covered more than 6 times more area than lesions in the

The usual American diet produced lesions covering more than 45 percent of the inner surface of the aorta while the prudent diet on the average produced lesions over only 7 percent of the aorta. Fig. 2 indicates that the percent of aortic surface involved with plaque was closely correlated with the serum cholesterol concentration.

The study also indicated that the fatty plaques resulting from the average American diet were four times more severe. The aortic lesions were studied microscopically in each animal by sampling constant standardized areas from each animal and assigning each lesion a number from one to four according to their severity – the worse the lesion, the higher the number. The total "severity numbers" in the eleven animals consuming the prudent diet was five. For the animals fed the average American diet, it was twenty-one.

Table I. Diet composition (average of 6 analyses) and food consumption

	AMERICAN AVERAGE		AMERICAN PRUDENT	
	DRY WT. %	CONSUMED GM/DAY	DRY WT. %	CONSUMED GM/DAY
FAT	22.6	26.9	18.0	14.0
PROTEIN	25.0	29.8	31.5	24.4
CARBOHYDRATES	45.6	54.3	44.5	34.5
CHOLESTEROL	136 mg	174.6 mg	90 mg	80.5 mg
ASH	2.2	2.6	2.5	1.9
FIBER	3.2	3.8	3.3	2.6
TOTAL SOLIDS	98.6	117.4	99.8	77.4
WATER GM/100 GM OF SOLIDS	101.4		150.0	
DAILY CALORIES/MONKEY		560		360
DAILY FOOD CONSUMP. (GM)		260.6		223.8

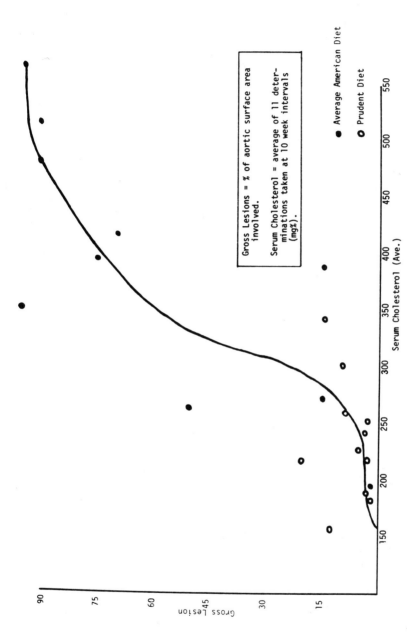

Fig. 2. The relationship between the average serum cholesterol concentration and the extent of aortic atheromatous lesions at autopsy (three experiments, each of two years duration, with human table-prepared diets).

A parallel part of the study dealth with the frequency and severity of lesions in the coronary arteries of the two groups. This
microscopic analysis showed that animals fed the average American
diet had more than four times as many coronary atherosclerotic lesions as the prudently fed animals - twenty-seven lesions versus
six lesions. The coronary artery lesions were also found to be
four times as severe in the average American-fed animals - the
"severity total" was nine for the typical diet and two for the
prudent American diet.

These studies offer a direct experimental demonstration in a
very good model of atherosclerosis in man that the table-prepared
average American ration results in the kind of arterial disease
that may increase the likelihood of heart attacks. It may be the
first laboratory investigation in which the foods found most frequently in the daily diet have been used in their usual proportions
and in the prepared form that they are usually consumed.

Fig. 2 shows a comparison of the extent of the lesions seen in
the aortas of each of these animals with the average serum cholesterol level each animal sustained throughout the study. It shows a
remarkable direct correlation in most of these animals. The sharp
upswing in severity or extent of aortic involvement with atherosclerosis when the serum cholesterol is maintained at 250 mg% or above
is similar (in agreement) to the results of numerous epidemiologic
studies in man.

The results of the study also support the theory that a moderate alteration of man's diet such as that recommended by the Report
of the Inter-Society Commission for Heart Disease Resources (30)
will inhibit the development of atherosclerosis.

A third type of dietary study for which the Rhesus monkey has
been successfully utilized is the demonstration of regression and
reversal of advanced atherosclerotic lesions. This has been done
by shifting the animals from a diet that is high in fat and high in
cholesterol and severely atherogenic to one that is either devoid
of or low in cholesterol and which is either very low in fat or has
polyunsaturated vegetable fat substituted for saturated fat and
which results in a very low blood cholesterol concentration.

The most fully developed of these studies is the one at the
University of Iowa (31,32,33). Armstrong, Connor, Warner and their
coworkers report that it is possible to produce severe aortic and
coronary artery disease in the Rhesus monkey in 17 months utilizing
a monkey ration enriched with eggs and other fatty foods to produce
a diet containing 41% fat and 1.2% cholesterol which in the monkey
sustains a serum cholesterol level of about 700 mg%. They were
able to lower these serum cholesterol levels to an average sustained concentration of less than 140 mg% either by feeding a low-fat,
low-cholesterol diet or by shifting the monkeys to a low cholesterol ration high in polyunsaturated fat. When either of these rations

were fed for 40 months then there was a remarkable decrease in severity of atherosclerosis so that coronary luminal narrowing was
reduced from 50-60% narrowing down to 15-20% narrowing. In general
the low-fat, low-cholesterol ration was slightly more effective
than the high polyunsaturated fat, low cholesterol diet.

We have just completed our first reversal experiment in the
Rhesus monkey. In this study we utilized our coconut oil-butter
fat cholesterol-containing ration which results, we believe, in an
accelerated atherogenesis. When fed for 73 weeks (14 months) this
ration consistently produced severe atherosclerosis in the aorta
and its main branches, including the coronary arteries. Although
we are still evaluating the results our study thus far indicates
that we have produced substantial regression in both coronary artery and aortic atherosclerosis. Not only does most of the lipid
disappear from these space occupying lesions but we have found, as
did Armstrong and coworkers (34) that the collagen content decreases substantially and there appears to be a real reduction in acid
mucopolysaccharide. The net result is that the real mass of the
lesions is greatly reduced and the large, soft, lipid-rich, atherosclerotic plaque is changed to a small, firm, smooth, slightly
elevated nodule which probably would never be of any clinical importance. We are busy planning future reversal experiments in
which we will test ways of treating the various types of lesions
we have been able to produce with various food fats.

ACKNOWLEDGEMENT

The authors wish to indicate their gratitude for the help of
Mr. Randolph Hughes in many technical aspects of the work that is
referred to in this paper and the assistance of Georgia Mohr and
Susan Thomas in preparing this manuscript.

REFERENCES

1. Gets, G.S., Vesselinovitch, D. and Wissler, R.W.
   A dynamic pathology of atherosclerosis.
   Am. J. Med. 46: 657, 1969.
2. Taylor, C.B., Cox, G.E., Manalo-Estrella, P. and
   Southworth, J.
   Atherosclerosis in Rhesus monkeys.
   A.M.A. Arch. Path. 74: 16, 1962.
3. Taylor, C.B., Manalo-Estrella, P. and Cox, G.E.
   Atherosclerosis in Rhesus monkeys. V. Marked
   diet-induced hypercholesteremia with xanthomatosis and
   severe atherosclerosis.
   A.M.A. Arch. Path. 76: 239, 1963.

4. Taylor, C.B., Patton, D.C. and Cox, G.E.
Atherosclerosis in Rhesus monkeys. VI. Fatal
myocardial infarction in a monkey fed fat and
cholesterol.
A.M.A. Arch. Path. 76: 404, 1963.
5. Wissler, R.W. and Vesselinovitch, D.
Differences between human and animal atherosclerosis.
Proceedings of the Third International Symposium on
Atherosclerosis.
In press, 1974.
6. Wissler, R.W. and Vesselinovitch, D.
Experimental models of human atherosclerosis.
Annals N.Y. Acad. Sci. 149: 907, 1968.
7. Nam, S.C., Lee, W. and Jarmolych, J.
Rapid production of advanced atherosclerosis in swine.
Fed. Proc. 32: 569abs, 1973.
8. Lee, K.T., Jarmolych, J., Kim, D.N., Grant, C., Krasney, J.A.,
Thomas, W.A. and Bruno, A.M.
Production of advanced coronary atherosclerosis, myocardial
infarction and "sudden death" in swine.
Exp. Mol. Path. 15: 170, 1971.
9. Luginbühl, H., Ratcliffe, H.L. and Detweiler, D.K.
Failure of egg-yolk feeding to accelerate progress of
atherosclerosis in older female swine.
Virchows Arch. Abt. A. Path. Anat. 348: 281, 1969.
10. Wissler, R.W.
Recent progress in studies of experimental primate
atherosclerosis. In: Progress in Biochemical Pharmacology,
vol. 4, p. 378. Miras, C.J., Howard, A.N. and Paoletti, R.,
eds. S. Karger, Basel/New York, 1968.
11. Wissler, R.W., Frazier, L.E., Hughes, R.H. and Rasmussen, R.A.
Atherogenesis in the Cebus monkey. I. A comparison of three
food fats under controlled dietary conditions.
A.M.A. Arch. Path. 74: 312, 1962.
12. Malmros, H. and Sternby, N.H.
Induction of atherosclerosis in dogs by a thiouracil free
semi-synthetic diet, containing cholesterol and hydrogenated coconut oil. In: Progress in Biochemical Pharmacology,
vol. 4, p. 482.
Miras, C.H., Howard, A.N. and Paoletti, R.,
eds. S. Karger, Basel/New York, 1968.
13. Robertson, A.L., Butkus, A., Ehrhart, L.A. and Lewis, L.A.
Experimental atherosclerosis in dogs. Evaluation of anatomopathological findings.
Atherosclerosis 15: 307, 1972.
14. Wissler, R.W., Vesselinovith, D., Getz, G.S. and Hughes, R.H.
Aortic lesions and blood lipids in Rhesus monkeys fed three
food fats.
Fed. Proc. 26: 2, 1967.

15. Vesselinovitch, D., Getz, G.S., Hughes, R. and Wissler, R.W.
    Coronary artery lesions in Rhesus monkeys fed corn oil,
    butter fat or peanut oil.
    Circulation, 46: 25abs, 1972.
16. Vesselinovith, D., Getz, G.S., Hughes, R.H. and Wissler, R.W.
    Atherosclerosis in the Rhesus monkey fed three fodd fats.
    Atherosclerosis.
    In press, 1974.
17. Kritchevsky, D., Tepper, S.A., Vesselinovitch, D. and
    Wissler, R.W.
    Cholesterol vehicle in experimental atherosclerosis.
    XI. Peanut oil.
    Atherosclerosis, 14: 53, 1971.
18. Kritchevsky, D., Tepper, S.A., Vesselinovitch, D and
    Wissler, R.W.
    Cholesterol vehicle in experimental atherosclerosis.
    XIII. Randomized peanut oil.
    Atherosclerosis 17: 225, 1973.
19. Gresham, G.A. and Howard, A.N.
    The independent production of atherosclerosis and thrombosis
    in the rat.
    Brit. J. Exp. Patch. 41: 395, 1960.
20. Scott, R.F., Morrison, E.S., Thomas, W.A., Jones, R. and
    Nam, S.C.
    Short-term feeding of unsaturated versus saturated fat
    in the production of atherosclerosis in the rat.
    J. Exp. Mol. Path., 3: 421, 1964.
21. Scott, R.F., Jones, R., Daoud, A.S., Zumbo, O.,
    Coulston, F. and Thomas, W.A.
    Experimental atherosclerosis in Rhesus monkeys. II. Cellular
    elements of proliferative lesions and possible role of cyto-
    plasmic degeneration in pathogenesis as studied by electron-
    microscopy.
    J. Exp. Mol. Path., 7: 34, 1967.
22. Florentin, R.A. and Nam, S.C.
    Dietary-induced atherosclerosis in miniature swine.
    I. Gross and light microscopy observations:
    Time of development and morphologic characteristics of lesions.
    J. Exp. Mol. Path., 8: 263, 1968.
23. Imai, H., Lee, K.T., Pastori, S., Panlilio, E.,
    Florentin, R. and Thomas, W.A.
    Atherosclerosis in rabbits.
    J. Exp. Mol. Path., 5: 273, 1966.
24. Thomas, W.A., Jones, R., Scott, R.F., Morrison, E.,
    Goodale, F. and Imai, H.
    Production of early atherosclerotic lesions in rats
    characterized by proliferation of modified smooth
    muscle cells.
    J. Exp. Mol. Path., Suppl. 1: 40, 1963.

25. Kritchevsky, D. and Tepper, S.A.
    Factors affecting atherosclerosis in rabbits fed
    cholesterol free diet.
    Life Sciences, 4: 1467, 1965.
26. Butkus, A., Robertson, A.L., Ehrhart, L.A. and Lewis, L.A.
    Aortic lipids at different stages of canine experimental
    arteriosclerosis.
    Exp. Mol. Path., 16: 311, 1972.
27. Wissler, R.W., Hughes, R.H., Frazier, L.E., Getz, G.S.
    and Turner, D.
    Aortic lesions and blood lipids in Rhesus monkeys fed
    "table-prepared" human diets.
    Circulation, 32: 220abs, 1965.
28. Wissler, R.W., Vesselinovitch, D., Hughes, R.,
    Turner, D. and Frazier, L.E.
    Atherosclerosis and blood lipids in Rhesus monkeys
    fed human table-prepared diets.
    Circulation, 44: 57abs, 1971.
29. Wissler, R.W.
    Development of the atherosclerotic plaque.
    Hospital Practice, 8: 61, 1973.
30. Stamler, J. et al.
    Primary prevention of the atherosclerotic diseases.
    Report of Inter-Society Commission for Heart Disease Resources.
    Circulation, 42: A-84, 1970.
31. Armstrong, M.L., Warner, D.E. and Connor, W.E.
    Regression of coronary atheromatosis in Rhesus monkeys.
    Circulation, 39: 2, 1969.
32. Armstrong, M.L., Warner, D.E. and Connor, W.E.
    Regression of coronary atheromatosis in Rhesus monkeys.
    Circ. Res., 27: 59, 1970.
33. Armstrong, M.L. and Megan, M.B.
    Nature of arterial lipid depletion in regression of
    experimental coronary atheromas in Rhesus monkeys.
    Circulation, 42: 35, 1970.
34. Armstrong, M.L. and Megan, M.B.
    Arterial fibrous proteins in Cynomolgus monkeys after
    atherogenic and regression regimens.
    Circulation, 48: 41abs, 1973.

DRUGS AND FOODS ON CONTRACTION OF ENDOTHELIAL CELLS AS A KEY
MECHANISM IN ATHEROGENESIS AND TREATMENT OF ATHEROSCLEROSIS WITH
ENDOTHELIAL-CELL RELAXANTS (CYCLIC AMP PHOSPHODIESTERASE INHIBITORS)

T. SHIMAMOTO

Institute for Cardiovascular Diseases, Tokyo Ika-Shika

National University Medical School, Tokyo, Japan

Sixty years have passed since Anitschkow succeeded in producing an atheroma in his experiment by "cholesterol loading" in
rabbits. Until the author (1972)(31,33) the mechanism of a atherogenesis remained unresolved as a long time enigma.

It has been found by us that the endothelial cells of internal lining of the arteries exhibit a contracting and swallowing
reaction immediately following Anitschkow's one shot treatment
with cholesterol in rabbits, although the active agent responsible
for the response remained unknown. We have named this phenomenon
"endothelial cell contraction". The contraction of the endothelial
cells results in enlargement of the intercellular space, thus allow-
ing penetration of relatively large particles of serum components
such as beta-lipoprotein (150-250A in diameter) into the subendothelial layer via the widened intercellular space channel and ac-
tivates at the same time the membrane flows and vesiculation for
the large particles by the contraction.

That the migration and subsequent deposition of beta-lipoprotein and pre-beta-lipoprotein into the subendothelial layer lead
to the formation of atheroma is today textbook knowledge, but the
"how" of this infiltrative mechanism had been an unanswered question
(11) until the author (1972). Here, it is noteworthy as shown by
us(31-33) that the endothelial cell contraction can also be caused
by the hitherto well known drugs and foods that can induce the so-
called edematous arterial reaction (26) and some of such substances
were also shown to induce the contraction by Robertson et al. (23)
independently from the author. Such active substances include various vaso-active substances such as epinephrine, norepinephrine,
angiotensinII serotonin, bradykinin, etc. or cholesterol, animal
fats, and several saturated fatty acids.

77

Based on the new findings aforementioned (Activation of the contracting and swallowing activity of endothelial cell - penetration of lipid particles into the subendothelial layer), we have been able to formulate a new concept in terms of prevention and treatment of atherosclerosis (25,31).

EPIDEMIOLOGIC STUDIES OF ATHEROSCLEROSIS
FACTS AND ACHIEVEMENTS

There is no doubt at this time that a clear-cut correlation exists between the severity of atherosclerosis and the incidence of heart attack as well as stroke. Stamler et al. (1972) (8) has pointed out that the progression of atherosclerosis is significantly related to 3 major risk factors. These are (1) hypercholesterolemia (2), hypertension and (3) cigarette smoking. As far as the atherosclerotic coronary artery disease goes, the risk factors were found to contribute alone or in combination to morbidity and mortality of myocardial infarction. Similar facts were confirmed in postmortem study of the severity of atherosclerosis as related to these three risk factors. The progress of cerebral atherosclerosis of Japanese has been shown to be faster than that of American by Resch et al. (1967)(32) despite the lower serum cholesterol level of Japanese than American. However, the hypertension is actually quite high in its incidence among Japanese under the habit of their characteristically high salt diet.

WHAT QUESTIONS ARE TO BE ANSWERED ?

The result of the emidemiologic (8) study tells us that, among the risk factors, hypercholesterolemia alone demonstrated no specific relation to atherosclerosis. Each of the 3 factors bears equivalent weight in pathogenesis, and when two or three factors were combined, synergistic relationship was found in terms of progression of atherosclerosis and in particular, of incidence of myocardial infarction. In another word, the people without hypercholesterolema very often suffer from a quite severe atherosclerosis. Why? This question must be answered first.

Laragh (18) and Kaneko (14) reported that among hypertensive diseases, one associated with low blood level of renin has good prognosis and least incidence of heart attack or stroke. These findings are important enough requiring further investigation to elucidate the linkage between renin-angiotensin system and progression of atherosclerosis.

It has been suspected until recently that neutral fats together with cholesterol had shares in producing atherosclerosis, but current lines of investigations have revealed facts contrary to this assumption (12). Epidemiological studies (16) show that it is rather hyperlipidemia with beta-lipoprotein and pre-beta-lipoprotein (Type 2,3,4,5 after Fredrickson) that accounts for atherosclerosis. Why is this certain type of hyperlipidemia associated with the progression of atherosclerosis?

One exceptional case gives us a clue. It is of extreme interest to note that again the epidemiological study (16) has shown us that in families with Type 1 hyperlipoproteinemia, there are few atherosclerotic cases, and practically, no progression of atherosclerotic lesions can be detected among these families (16). It is almost incredible to learn about this fact; that patients who suffer from Type 1 hyperlipoproteinemia, who carry extremely high level of lipids, quite often inclusive of cholesterol, whose condition is life-long because of genetic trait, can be minimally attacked by atherosclerotic process. One would have to give an answer that accounts for this striking phenomenon.

BRIEF SUMMARY OF OUR FINDINGS

The beginning of our atherosclerosis research dates back to many years ago when we had confirmed a peculiar edematous reaction occuring on the internal lining of the arterial wall of rabbits and rhesus monkeys whenever the animals had been treated with atherogenic substances. We termed this phenomenon "edematous arterial reaction" (26). Among atherogenic substances those that are definitively producing atheroma like in the case of repetitive administration of cholesterol have been categorized into one group while the others including epinephrine and angiotensin II have been placed into another category which was deemed to be responsible for the progression of atherosclerosis. Needless to say angiotensin II is also an active agent in renal hypertension and epinephrine is also an active agent in cigarette smoking. In either case, rabbits and rhesus monkeys treated with these substances all showed "edematous arterial reaction" (26) , while rats, non susceptible animal to atherosclerosis, showed almost no or a minimal such a reaction. We then have come to recognize that the edematous arterial reaction is nothing but a part of complex and integral chain reaction involving both the arterial wall and the blood component, especially platelets, in terms of changes in morphology as well as physico-chemical properties, and the reaction is always accompanied by thrombogenic tendency (26). The fact that acid mucopolysaccharides appear in the edematous portion of the arterial wall (26) and that it has an extreme resemblance to the pathologically defined pattern of early stage atherosclerosis have motivated us to delve deeper into this topic at that time.

As will be described in detail later, we have been fortunate in discovering the substances that can prevent or offset the said edematous arterial reaction (26) at a relatively earlier stage of our investigation. Pyridinolcarbamate (PDC) is the one which was found to be one of the above "preventive substances" (16). This agent (PDC) has been shown to be effective in the prevention of

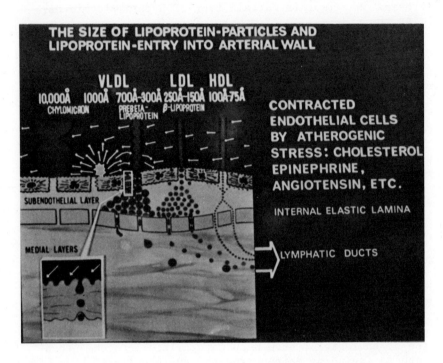

Fig. 1. This figure shows the passage of large particles of the plasma, like beta-lipoprotein or pre-beta-lipoprotein, through the endothelial lining into the subendothelial space and through small holes of the internal elastic lamina and into the media.

By the contracting and swallowing activity of stimulated endothelial cells, namely by widening of the intercellular junctions and by their activated membrane flow or membrane vesiculation, it is possible for large particles with the size of beta- and pre-beta-lipoproteins, to enter the subendothelial space from the blood stream through the endothelial lining. However, it seems impossible for chylomicron, because of their too large size.

Beta-lipoprotein is large enough to be delayed in passing through holes of the internal elastic lamina. Especially larger groups of lipoproteins such as Lp(a), flating beta-lipoprotein and pre-beta-lipoprotein, the passage through the endothelial lining may certainly be possible, but the further passage through such small holes of the internal elastic lamina seems highly difficult, because carbon particles with almost the same size with these lipoproteins enter easily the subendothelial space, but they were almost impossible to pass through the internal elastic lamina and remained there over months. Such facts may suggest the atherogenic mechanism.

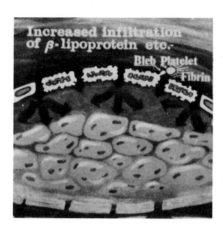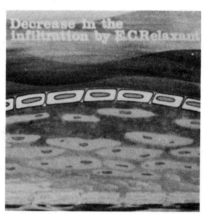

Fig. 2. Contraction and Blebbing of Endothelial Cells Covering
Atheroma Treatment with Endothelial Cell Relaxant.

The left picture shows that the contracting activity of endothelial cells enlarges the intercellular space and increases the
membrane flow and vesiculation inducing penetration of cholesterol-
bearing large lipoproteins from the blood stream into the subendothelial space. This results in the stagnation of cholesterol-bear-
ing lipoproteins leading to formation of atheromatous lesions in
the subendothelial space (left). The right picture shows that re-
laxation of endothelial cells reduces the size of intercellular
space and inhibits the membrane flow and vesculation, which in turn,
inhibits or reduces the infirltration of large plasma particles
through the intercellular space into the subendothelial space, thus
exhibiting the curative effect of endothelial-cell relaxant.

        E.C. : Endothelial-cell
        F.C. : Foam Cells

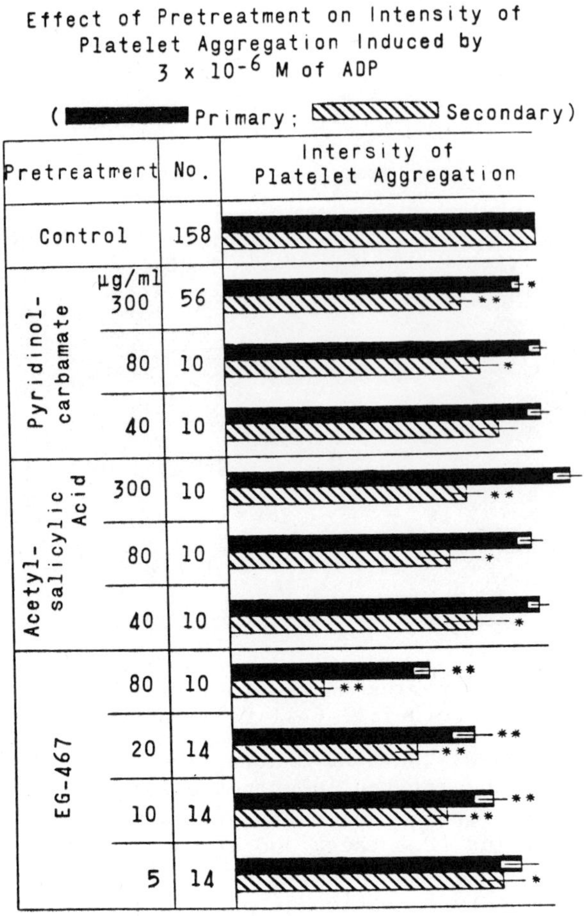

Effect of Pretreatment on Intensity of
Platelet Aggregation Induced by
3×10^{-6} M of ADP

(� Primary; ▨▨▨▨▨ Secondary)

Fig. 3. Human platelets, suspended in citrated platelet rich
plasma, were incubated with the saline solution with different
concentration of PDC or aspirin or EG467, and as a control, with
saline for 5 minutes at 37 C, and, then, were undergone the measurement of ADP-induced platelet-aggregability by optical density method (Didisheim, P., Sturm, R.E. and Owen, Jr., C.A.: Experiments
on Thrombosis and its Prevention. Current Concepts of Coagulation
and Hemostasis. p. 177-185, 1971 F.K. Schattaner Verlag, Stuttgart-
New York).
Note: The primary aggregation of platelets is significantly inhibited by PDC and EG467, but not by acetylsalicylic acid, while
the secondary aggregation is inhibited by all these substances.
Highly potent inhibitory effect of EG467 is noted.

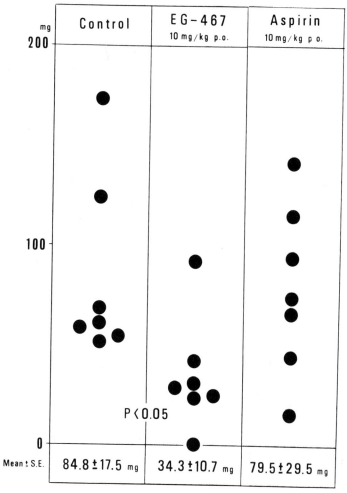

Fig. 4.   The carotid artery of rabbit was connected to polyethylene tube and its another end was connected to the other side of jugular vein and the vein was narrowed at two positions at its central parts. Thus the thrombus was produced at the end of polyethylene tube in the venous lumen and the preventive effect of certain drug on the formation thrombus was evaluated by the weight of thrombus formed (Kurai, A.: Ochanomizu Med. J. 13: 199, 1965).

Note: This figure shows the preventive effect of EG467 (10 mg/kg p.o.).

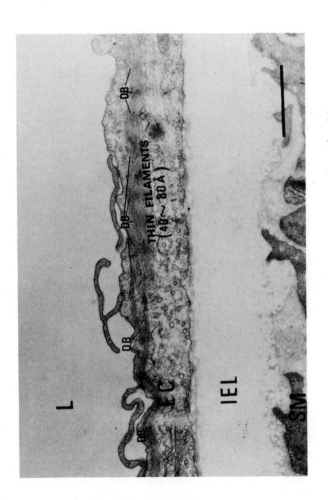

Photo 1.   Endothelial cell of rabbit aorta transected longitudinally.
(1)   Note: Longitudinally running thin filaments with dense bodies (D) are seen.
          The dense bodies well correspond with the concaved parts of the endothelial surface.
              L : Lumen   D: Dense body   EC: Endothelial cell
            IEL: Internal elastic lamina   SM: Smooth muscle

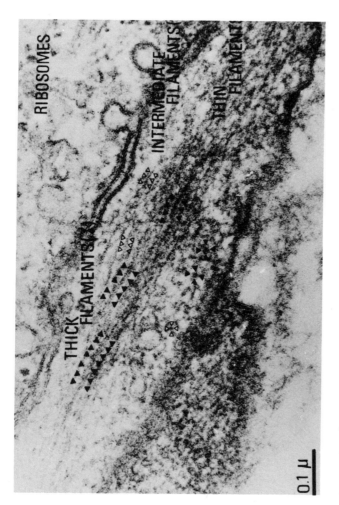

Photo 1.   Endothelial cell of rabbit aorta transected longitudinally.
(2)   Note: Thick filaments are seen among thin filaments showing the resemblance to
those of smooth muscle cells. Intermediate filaments are also seen apart from
this filament.

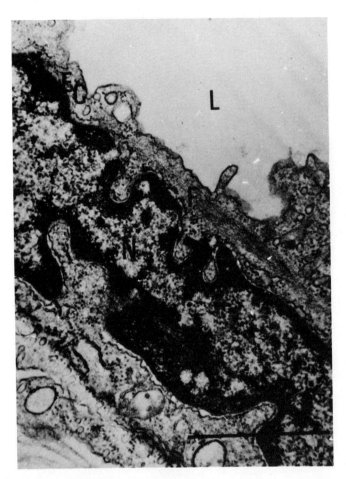

Photo 2.   Endothelial cells of thoracic aorta of rabbit samples
2 hours after cholesterol challenge (1 g/kg p.o.).

Note: The nucleus shows strong indentations and pinch (↑) formation.
In the neighbouring cytoplasm of the pinch, many thin filaments (F)
are seen running longitudinally and are considered to be the contracting actomyosin responsible for the formation of pinch.

       L: Aortic lumen   EC: Endothelial cell
       N: Nucleus   F :   Thin filaments

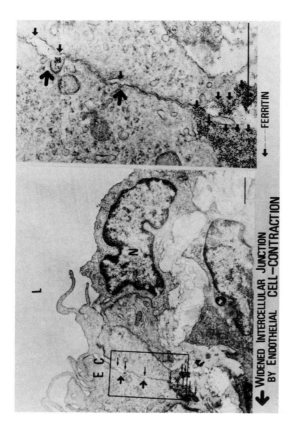

Photo 3. Transection of the intima of thoracic aorta of a rabbit receiving angiotensin II, iμg:kg i.v. and ferritin, 700 mg i.v. as a marker, 10 minutes thereafter. This specimen was sampled following a vital fixation of the aorta which had been performed 10 minutes after an intravenous injection of ferritin.

Note: Ferritin particles are passing through the intercellular space from the aortic lumen to the subendothelial space. They are seen as widened area (↑) in the intercellular space and at its orificium area (↑) in the subendothelial space.

L: Aortic lumen   EC: Endothelial cell   N: Nucleus

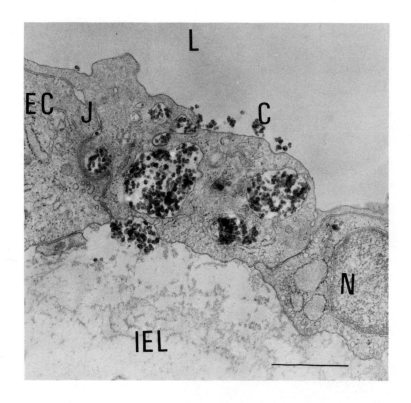

Photo 4. Electron microscopic picture of the transection of the
intima of thoracic aorta of the rabbit, which was challenged by
carbon particles (50% Pelikan ink 5 ml/kg i.v.) and angiotensin II
(10 µg/kg i.v.) and was sacrificed 30 minutes after the challenge.

Note: Carbon particles are passing through the cytoplasm and intercellular junction into the subendothelial space by contracting and
swallowing activity of the endothelial cells activated by the challenge.

            L : Aortic lumen   C: Carbon particles
            EC : Endothelial cell   J: Intercellular junction
            IEL: Internal Elastic lamina N: Nucleus

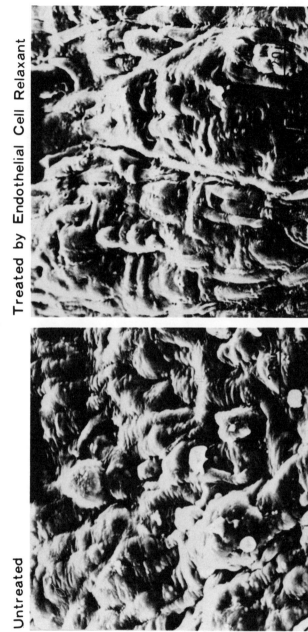

Untreated

Treated by Endothelial Cell Relaxant

Many horizontal lines represent the contraction of endothelial cells.

Horizontal lines have been markedly reduced by pyridinolcarbamate (10mg/kg p.o. given 2hrs. before sacrifice.)

Photo 5.   Scanning electron microscopic picture of the endothelial cells covering atheroma.   -   In Cholesterol-fed rabbits   -

Note: Untreated (left): Many horizontal wrinkles represent the contraction of endothelial cells.

Treated by endothelial cell relaxant (right): Horizontal wrinkles have been markedly reduced by pyridinolcarbamate (10 mg/kg p.o. given 2 hours before sacrifice).

Photo 6. Scanning electron microscopic demonstration of endothelial cell-contraction

(1) Angiotensin II side   (2) Saline side

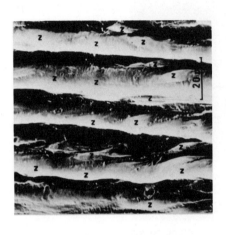

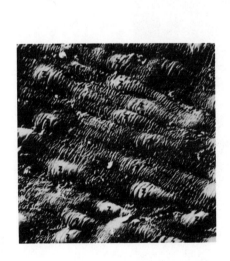

The both common carotid arteries were temporarily clamped and the saline or 10 mg/ml of angiotensin II were separately injected into their lumen of the right carotid artery and the left carotid artery respectively at the peripheral part of the clamp and immediately after removing the clamps, the endothelial surface of (1) the left and (2) right carotid artery was simultaneously fixed by 2.5% glutaraldehyde through the catheter placed in the left ventricle.   CB: Cell Boundary

Note: (1) the angiotensin II side was fixed at a moderately vasodilative state. The boundaries of each endothelial cells are relatively clear and the vertical wrinkles of each endothelial cells were produced by contraction of the endothelial cells by angiotensin II and look like a washing board ("the washing board phenomenon"). They are considered to contribute to the increase in thrombogenic activity of platelets, because the wrinkles are just vertical to the direction of the blood flow. (2) The saline side: The surface of each endothelial cells is smooth, despite the moderate vasoconstrictive state with deep folds due to the contraction of arterial smooth muscles.

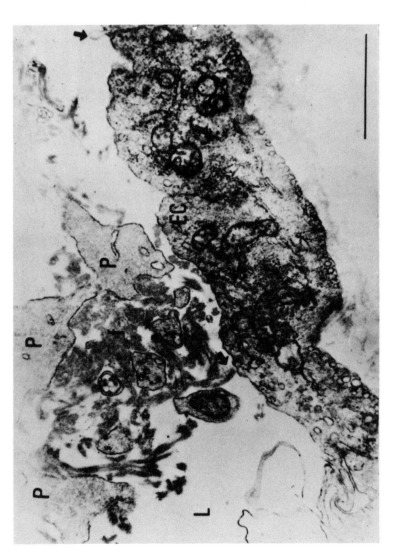

Photo 7. Transection of the intima of thoracic aorta of rabbits received angiotensin II (10 µg/kg i.v.) 30 minutes before the sampling of this specimen.

Note: A part of endothelial cells with blebs (↑). Left one is stuck by platelets, around which fibrin had been formed.

L: Aortic lumen   P: Platelet   f: Fibrin   EC: Endothelial cell   Arrow: Bleb

Table I. Contraction of Endothelial Cells

Challenge	Pretreatment	T E M			Immunofluorescent antibody technique	
		Number of animals	Number of EC counted	Pinches	Number of animals	Infiltration of β-lipoprotein
No	No	10	934	0	7	- ~ ±
Cholesterol, 1 g/kg p.o.	No	10	972	6.2 ± 1.1^{c}	7	$+++^{a}$
	Premarin, 5 mg/kg i.v.	5	526	0	3	- ~ ±
	PDC, 10 mg/kg p.o.	5	548	0	5	- ~ ±
Epinephrine, 1 µg/kg i.v.	Placebo	5	536	4.1 ± 1.2^{b}	5	$+++^{a}$
	PDC, 10 mg/kg p.o.	5	520	0	5	- ~ ±
Angiotensin II, 1 µg/kg i.v.	Placebo	7	453	4.3 ± 1.2^{b}	5	$+++^{a}$
	PDC, 10 mg/kg p.o.	6	510	0	5	- ~ ±
Bradykinin, 10 µg/kg i.v.	Placebo	6	520	2.7 ± 1.0^{b}	5	$+++^{a}$
	PDC, 10 mg/kg p.o.	6	515	0	5	- ~ ±
Serotinin, 10 µg/kg i.v.	Placebo	5	486	5.4 ± 1.8^{c}	5	$+++^{a}$
	PDC, 10 mg/kg p.o.	5	503	0	5	- ~ ±

PDC : Pyridinolcarbamate;

Control vs Challenged -- [a] $p < 0.5$; [b] $p < 0.1$; [c] $p < 0.001$.

Table II.   Follow-up Study on Patients Suffering from
            Arteriosclerosis Obliterans under Pyridinol-
            carbonate Treatment and other Treatment

	Pyridinolcarbamate group	Nonpyridinolcarbamate group
Total number of patients	45	60
Age (years)	50.7 ± 2.4	53.0 ± 1.5
History of disease (months)	50.0 ± 10.9	48.9 ± 6.8
Severity of disease		
Type II	39	57
Type IV	6	3
Blood cholesterol level		
(mg/dl)	198.8 ± 8.7	187.2 ± 5.2
Blood pressure (mm Hg)		
Systolic	149.4 ± 5.0	152.9 ± 5.1
Diastolic	83.5 ± 2.7	90.4 ± 2.4
Complications		
Diabetes mellitus	6	4
Myocardial infarction	2	2
Observation period (weeks)	211.5 ± 17.4	165.4 ± 13.0
Number of deaths by apoplectic		
and heart attacks	0	8*
Apoplectic attacks	1	2
Heart attacks	0	6

*$p < 0.05$.

(Atsumi, T., Honda, Y., and Matsuda, M.:   J. Jap. Coll. Angiol., in press)

the following experimentally induced atherosclerotic conditions;
(a) atheroma in the rabbit produced by cholesterol loading (32,38),
(b) arteriosclerosis induced by calciferol loading (10), (c) arteriosclerosis due to experimental lathyrism (39) and (d) diabetic
angiopathy and nephropathy of K.K. mice (6). It is also the first
so-called platelet drug used widely as an antithrombotic agent in
the history of medicine. Bearing all of the above findings in our
minds, we have reached the conclusion that, whatever may be the
cause, the key portion of atherogenesis lies in the edematous arterial reaction (26) in which triggering mechanism that leads to
full blown atherosclerosis is concealed.

In 1971, we were able to demonstrate the presence of serum
beta-lipoprotein in the edematous parts of aortic wall showing
the edematous arterial reaction (25,29,34). Namely just a few
hours after a single dose treatment of animals with cholesterol,
particles like beta-lipoprotein with diameters between 150-250A
infiltrated into the intima and further down to the media. The
mode of infiltration was such that the particles entered the subendothelial space first, temporarily dammed by the internal elastic
lamina, then into the muscular layers via pores in the internal
elastic lamina, and eventually have been carried away possibly
through lymphatic channels (25,29,34). The PDC has proved itself
to sufficiently reduce or prevent this infiltrative process to occur (25,34). At this juncture, we were faced upon with the underlying mechanism that can possibly provide an explanation as to why
the large particles such as beta-lipoprotein could be transported
into the subendothelial layer so rapidly that is almost instantaneous.

Studies on the Contracting and Swallowing Activity of the Endothelial Cells

In our laboratory, investigation dealing with the problem of
endothelial cell contraction was initiated in 1971. A catheter was
introduced into the left ventricle of rabbit under anesthesia,
through which perfusion of the fixative solution was carried out
under constant pressure (110 mmHg) in order to achieve direct in
situ fixation of the aortic endothelial cells. The fixative was
composed of 2.5% glutaraldehyde, isotonic, pH 7.4 with phosphate
buffer. In starting the perfusion, the said fixative warmed to
room temperature was used. The temperature was then rapidly lowered to ice-cold during the procedure. The specimen obtained in
this fashion was finally subjected to electron microscopic study.

The presence of contractile protein in the endothelial cells
has been known since Becker and Murphy (1969) (3,4) and among various contractile proteins, the presence of thin filaments (40-
90A) with dense bodies and thick filaments (130-160A) and of intermediate filaments (70-120A) were easily recognized in the endo-

thelial cells of rabbit and monkey. As a result of contraction, the nucleus shrinks down, forming indentations at its periphery. When actomyosin contracts vigorously, hollow formation becomes extreme to such a degree that both poles at the ceiling of the hollow could be seen in conjunction. Majno (1969) (20) referred to this phenomenon as "pinch", and we have used appearance and number of pinch and also indentations of nuclei as index of the endothelial cell contraction. We have also measured the size of interendothelial cellular space.

The results were as follows: in a group of rabbits used for control we were unable to observe any "pinch" phenomenon nor an enlargement of the intercellular space. The same was true with another group fed with placebo. To further demonstrate that no enlargement of the intercellular space and taken place, we gave ferritin by i.v. bolus, but no appearance of ferritin has been observed in the intercellular space and a few was seen in the sub-endothelial layer.

On the contrary, in a group of 10 rabbits who were given cholesterol (1 g/kg p.o.), who then killed one to two hours later, about 6.2% of their aortic endothelial cells exhibited "pinch" of the nucleus indicating the strong endothelial cell contraction. Similar findings were obtained with rabbits treated with epinephrine, angiotensin II, bradykinin, serotonin and prostaglandin E-1. The degree of enlargement of the interendothelial cellular space can sometimes reach 300A in diameter, although the enlargement was usually seen as localized ones scattered interruptedly along the cellular junction. Occasionally, we could see a localized enlargement measuring up to 900A in diameter. When ferritin or carbon particles (200-500A) was given on top of cholesterol or other above named substances, it appeared as clusters in the intercellular space. As shown in Photo. 4, the ferritin can be seen as scattered small clusters along the course of intercellular space, and at its opening into the subendothelial layer, there appears large aggregates of ferritin despite of scantiness of ferritin particles in vesicles at this stage. As shown in Photo. 5, carbon particles also passed the course of the intercellular space into the subendothelial layer. The membrane flow (Bennett 1956) and membrane vesiculation through cytoplasm was also activated in the later stage in the case of carbon transportation by the above mentioned challenge, when the contraction of the endothelial cell was extremely strongly induced, and the enhancement of membrane flow and membrane vesiculation seemed to be induced also by contracting activity of the endothelial cells.

Interrelationship between the Size of Lipoprotein, Endothelial Cell Contraction with Subsequent Enlargement of the Intercellular Space, and Transportation of the Lipid Particles.

Speaking of the enlargement of the intercellular space again, we have observed that the largest enlargement can be obtained after injection of angiotensin II. In the case of cholesterol, a considerable enlargement is usually elicited with upper limit of the range at 300-360A. The enlargement of the intercellular space can reach 700A, although rarely. Naturally, with this degree of enlargement, one can easily deduce that the small particles up to beta-lipoprotein (150-250A) could enter into the subendothelial layer with relative ease, and the intercellular route seems to be the main route for smaller particles, although the vesicle system and membrane flow for ferritin transportation were also activated by the above mentioned challenges. It is not impossible, if not always, for the larger particles of pre-beta-lipoprotein (300-700A) to enter through enlarged intercellular space, and the entry by membrane flow may be possible for pre-beta-lipoprotein as in the case of carbon particles, when endothelial cells are strongly activated as in the case of carbon entry. As far as chylomicron is concerned, its passage through the enlarged intercellular space is considered difficult, since the maximum enlargement we have ever observed was in the range of 900A in diameter, and this was only with the exceptional cases, and even its passage through cytoplasm by membrane flow is also difficult to be considered because of its large size.

Haust and more have stated in their recent book (1972) (11) : "It is nowadays widely accepted that once invasion of beta-lipoprotein and pre-beta-lipoprotein into the subendothelial layer occurs atherosclerosis can be eventually formulated through chain reactions. The mechanism of this invasion is not clear". In this context, our findings have shown a clue to the solution of enigma for all those who have been and are in the research of atherosclerosis.

Studies Using Immunofluorescence Method

As stated previously, the beta-lipoprotein invades into the arterial wall immediately following a single dose treatment of test animals with cholesterol, epinephrine or angiotensin II (25, 29,34). This finding was obtained with the use of immunofluorescence method.

Of extreme interest at this juncture is our finding with the rhesus monkey. In monkeys, for the beta-lipoprotein to further invade into the muscular zone after passing through the subendothelial layer as well as pores of internal elastic lamina, it takes a relatively longer time as compared with that of immunoglobulin G (IgG). There is a 30 minutes to one hour time delay in the case of beta-lipoprotein. This implies, at least as one possibility, that particles with the size of beta-lipoprotein could hardly penetrate through the internal elastic lamina, and therefore, tend to stagnate in the subendothelial layer, although there may be another explanation concerning the physical or chemical property of the particles. However, it is worthwhile to note that in the case of ferritin particle, the

transportation through the holes of internal elastic lamina was
performed just one by one. For carbon particles with the size of
pre-beta-lipoprotein, the passage through internal elastic lamina
is almost impossible and their stagnation in the subendothelial
space is marked taking at least over months, when carbon particles
once penetrate the endothelial lining. With the increase of particle size such as in the case of large beta-lipoprotein, floating
beta-lipoprotein and pre-beta-lipoprotein, the situation is deemed
to become more realistic, although, at this time, we do not have
the experimental data yet. Here, the reason why men with high
blood levels of beta- and pre-beta-lipoprotein are more prone to
atherosclerosis, could well be explained on the basis of above
findings. The toxicity of Lp(a) also may have a relationship to
the larger size of Lp(a) than beta-lipoprotein.

While, the fact that the cholesterol content of beta-lipoprotein is as high as 40%, is in itself significant, the very cause
of atheroma formation lies in the stagnation of lipoproteins in
the subendothelial layer, particularly due to the difficulty for
beta-lipoprotein and pre-beta-lipoprotein to further penetrate
downwards through the internal elastic lamina.

In the case of Type 1 hyperlipoproteinemia in which chylomicron constitutes the major carrier of cholesterol in the blood,
we would assume that atherosclerosis could seldom occur merely because of the large size of chylomicron particles (1,000-10,000A).
This is because, as stated before, the widening of the intercellular space secondary to the contraction of endothelial cells can,
at the most, reach only 900A and the membrane flow is almost impossible to carry such large particles.

Endothelial Cells Covering the Atheromatous Lesions
- Their Contraction and Relaxation -

When we studied the endothelial cells covering the atheroma
in experimentally induced atheromatous rabbits, we were able to
confirm that the "pinch" indicative of cell contraction appeared
in 6.2% of all endothelial cell observed, that there was concomitant of the interendothelial cellular space, and enhancement of
the membrane flow (Bennett) and membrane vesiculation, and that
ferritin and carbon particles were easily detectable on electron
micrograph in a fashion already mentioned. These facts fit the
finding of Lofland and Clarkson (1970) (19), who showed the increased influx of labelled cholesterol in atheromatous lesions as compared with the unaffected area. Administration of PDC or EG467 or
Premarin by mouth to such animals in a sufficient dose showed a
statistically significant decrease of the percentage of pinch appearance, and the pharmacological study of the same data revealed
statistically significant therapeutic effect of PDC on atherosclerotic lesions. When the PDC dose was increased to 30mg/kg, or the

animals were given EG467 1 mg/kg p.o. or Premarin 5 mg/kg i.v.,
cells showing the pinch have completely disappeared. In other
words, the above three substances exhibited a strong relaxing action
on the contracting and swallowing activity of endothelial cells.

What then have we considered was the possibility that insofar
as the widened intercellular space is narrowed, and the membrane
flow is limited, and infusion of lipoprotein be blocked, there
should follow infusions of only physiologic particles together with
water into the atheromatous lesion. Could it be conceivably admitted when we state that physiologic perfusion would help the repair
process of the diseased focus. In fact, the ongoing pharmacological
study (27) in our laboratory dealing with the effect of long term
administration of PDC, EG467 or Premarin to the atheromatous rabbits has already shown indication of healing of the atheroma which
is statistically significant in terms of acceleration rate of the
healing process. For the sake of simplicity, we give the general
term of "endothelial cell relaxants" to substances such as PDC,
EG467 and Premarin. The criterion of the therapeutic effect of
endothelial cell relaxants may well be established on the following
bases: it relaxes the endothelial cells; can decrease or block the
contraction of endothelial cells as well as subsequent enlargement
of the intercellular space and enhancement of the membrane flow
(this chain reaction is usually caused by the activator substances
of 3 major risk factors such as cholesterol, epinephrine, angiotensin II, bradykinin, serotonin, histamine, prostaglandin E-1 and
some causative agents of inflammation); and eventually displays the
vital effect of preventing infusion of beta-lipoprotein and pre-beta-
lipoprotein into the subendothelial space. It appears that, based
on the above mentioned preventive as well as therapeutic effect of
the endothelial cell relaxants, the prevention of atherosclerosis
is not unfeasible, and that, treatment of the established atheroma
could be facilitated. At this juncture, it is noteworthy that recent enzymatic studies covering these areas have proven positive
biochemical aspects of PDC in favour of its preventive and therapeutic effect on atherosclerosis. Numano et al. (1971) (21), (1973)
(41) reported that PDC has activated enzymes referrable to the re-
pairing process of atheroma, while Kritchevsky and Tepper (1971)
(15) demonstrated enhancement of cholesterol oxidation by PDC.
These new biochemical aspects of endothelial relaxants will of course, play on supplemental and complemental roles in our understanding
of the mechanism of atherogenesis and its treatment.

Interrelationship between the Endothelial Cell
Contraction and Thrombus Formation

The linkage between endothelial cell contraction and thrombus
formation is an important problem. When the endothelial cell goes
into extreme contraction by whatever the cause - cholesterol, epinephrine, angiotensin II, etc., - its ultrastructural appearance on

electron microscopy is characterized by the formation of vertical
wrinkles due to contraction of the longitudinally running actomyosin. We call this phenomenon "the washing board phenomenon",
because of its similarity. These winkles may undoubtedly induce
the turbulence of peripheral blood flow and tend to accelerate the
morphological and functional changes of platelets being responsible
for the increase in platelet-aggregability. In addition, the strong
contraction of the endothelial cells accompanies frequently formation of the blebs (30,34).In addition to this basic change, one
frequently sees sticking of the platelets to the blebs, and there
is usually a fibrin deposition. It seems to me that the part of
the cell membrane beneath which the bleb is formed is actually injured in such a way that the repelling ability against the platelet
has been lost. Losing the physiologic platelet repelling activity
the normal cell membrane tends to play a part in the aggregation
of platelets, thus leading to the fibrin formation. We have observed in the rabbits that whenever they were treated with a single dose of epinephrine, angiotensin II and/or cholesterol, there
has been transient increase of coagulability of the blood. Among
the mechanisms of this phenomenon, a serial reaction consisting of,
- injury of the platelet - its sticking and release serotonin, a
potent endothelial cell-contractor, and platelet factors - segre-
gation of stuck platelets to and from the part of qualitatively
altered cell membrane - recirculation of such segregated platelet-
aggregate into the blood stream (platelet-aggregability is now enhanced) - final increase of coagulability of the blood, was suggested. This type of chain reaction will probably repeat in a developing fashion resulting in formation as well as structural re-
inforcement of the atheromatous lesions.

        PDC (24,25) and EG467 (40) show direct effect on platelets of
both human and rabbits with the in vitro studies we were able to
demonstrate a strong inhibitory action of these agents against
the primary and secondary aggregations of platelets which had been
induced by ADP, epinephrine or collagen. In this regard, the
strength of PDC in terms of aggregation inhibition, was equivalent
to aspirin, whereas EG467 was more potent than aspirin and the effect of PDC and EG467 is roughly parallel to their potency as a cyclic AMP phosphodiesterase inhibitor.

        In the meantime, we looked into the preventive effect of PDC
(24,25) and EG467 (40) against the thrombogenic trend as well as
the increase of blood coagulability in rabbits who had been given
cholesterol, epinephrine and/or angiotensin II by one shot method.
These two agents showed a striking preventive effect against the
enhancement of coagulability and related thrombus formation. The
effective dose with PDC was 10 mg/kg, and 1 mg/kg with EG467. To
our surprise, however, the effective blood levels of these agents
were much lower than had been anticipated. In another words, it
was lower than in the case of in vitro study in which, as was mentioned before, investigation on the platelet aggregation and its

inhibition by PDC and EG467 were made. This finding of us is compatible with that of Cotton (1972) (7), who has observed the normalizing effect of PDC treatment on the elevated platelet-aggregability of patients suffering from severe arteriosclerosis obliterans, and their blood level of PDC was not enough high to lower directly the platelet-aggregability in vitro testing. At any rate, the fact that thrombosis contributes as a factor in the pathogenesis of atherosclerosis (8) has been well known to us now for more than two decades. When the pathologic section of atheromatous lesions is carefully examined one can often see the characteristic picture that symbolizes the formative process of atheroma. This includes sticking of the platelets to the arterial intima, and formation of thrombi which are frequently encapsulated by newly generated endothelial cells. Here, one may argue about the possible role of collagen as a factor giving rise to thrombus formation, for the endothelial cell contraction can also bring about exposure of the intercellular collagen tissue to the circulating blood by widening up the intercellular space. Of course, it may be important in the case of highly sensitive endothelial cells, to some contracting substances, but we feel that "the washing board phenomenon" by endothelial cell-contraction, the loss of platelet-repelling activity by the cell membrane due to injury or the blebbing caused by vigorous contraction may possible be significant as in the case of exposed collagen tissue.

USE OF ENDOTHELIAL CELL RELAXANTS AS THERAPEUTIC AGENT TO THE ATHEROSCLEROTIC DISEASES

It was in 1963 when first used PDC for treatment of atherosclerosis (28,35). Cerebral, coronary and peripheral atherosclerosclerosis have been chosen as major targets, and up till now, there are considerable numbers of reports as to the clinical trials on PDC from many countries all over the world (13,25,36) including Italy.

As regards prevention of cerebrovascular accident and/or myocardial infarction, I feel, on the basis of dialectics, that the use of endothelial cell relaxants as medicine deserves certain merit. Needless to say, willful removal or avoidance of various risk factors on the part of patients, combined with establishment of sound ecology is of primary importance but it sometimes takes too much time and often impossible so that the endothelial cell relaxants are required.

Especially in the prevention of arterial thrombosis, in which platelets and the endothelial surface play an essential role, PDC and EG467 exhibited a highly potent preventive effect in our experimental model of arterial thrombosis in rabbits. In man, Fukui tried PDC on as many as 4,083 patients who had survived strokes with resultant hemiplegias (9). These patients were divided into

two groups for the purpose of studying the frequency of recurrence
of stroke or development of myocardial infarction. One group was
treated with PDC, and the other which formed the control group was
treated otherwise. The PDC group showed lower incidence of both
recurrent stroke and myocardial infarction than did the other
group, which was statistically significant. Atsumi (2)   also carried out a similar study, but dealt with advanced cases of occlusive peripheral artery disease. All these patients had presented
either severe intermittent claudication of cyanosis of the lower
extremities with or without ischemic ulcers. Forty-five cases were given PDC and 60 cases were given other modality of therapy,
and that all were followed up for a period of 4 years. In PDC
group, none developed myocardial infarction and only one had a
stroke which he survived (P < 0.05). Among the control group, however, six had myocardial infarction and two had stroke, all succumb-
ed.

FUTURE PERSPECTIVE

        Up till this time, the atherosclerosis research has accumul-
ated great numbers of new knowledges regarding the relationship
between atherogenesis and lipid metabolism as well as enzymatic
processes involved therein. These new knowledges are of inestimable
value in our understanding of atherogenesis and the repair processes of arterial wall.

        However, at the present moment, it seems not unreasonable to
emphasize the importance of the efforts to further eludicate the
nature of contractile protein within the endothelial cells of the
arterial intima, and the relationship between the contraction and
the endogenous cyclic AMP level, which has been already established in various smooth muscles, because the cyclic AMP phosphodiesterase inhibiting activity has been shown to be quite high in PDC and
especially EG467. Also the current studies on the effects of endothelial cell relaxants on various vascular injuries must be expanded.

        Nevertheless, it seems to me that the current lines of study
on pathophysiology of the arterial endothelial cells, especially
of investigation of actomyosin and adenyl cyclase-Cyclic AMP-phos-
phodiesterase system of endothelial cells would soon become a new
and important field in cardiovascular research. In a way, the current status of atherosclerosis research is as specific and extensive as the one we had experienced in the past years with the topics of "hypertension versus actomyosin of arterial smooth muscle".
Recently the lowering of cyclic AMP in arteriolar smooth muscle is
thought to be a fundamental mechanism in elevation of hypertension.
Similarly the powerful preventive effect of cyclic AMP phosphodiesterase inhibitors such as PDC and the EG467 on the progress of atherosclerosis may suggest lowering of cyclic AMP in arterial endothelial cells as alpha an accerelating mechanism in atherogenesis,

which is to be elevated.

Conclusion. The contraction of endothelial cells, which induce the entry of large particles such as beta-lipoprotein (and
presumably pre-beta-lipoprotein) into the subendothelial space and,
at the same time, the enhancement of thrombogenic activity of the
blood, especially of platelets, seems to be the key mechanism in
atherogenesis and thrombogenesis. For the prevention and treatment of atherosclerosis, the above mentioned our findings may suggest the importance of three active procedures besides the removal
of risk factors. (1) The inhibition and reduction of the entry
of beta-lipoprotein and pre-beta-lipoprotein into the subendothelial space in all atherosclerotic conditions with or without hyper-
proteinemia by the endothelial cell relaxant, which inhibits at
the same time the sticking and aggregating activity of platelets.
(33).The elevation of abnormally lowered Cyclic AMP in the arterial
endothelial cells. (34) The lowering and normalizing of beta-lipoprotein and pre-beta-lipoprotein of the blood, instead of simple
hypocholesterolemic procedure, in cases with elevated beta- and
pre-beta-lipoprotein.

REFERENCES

1. Anitschkow, N.N.: Über die Veränderungen der Kaninchenaorta
   bei experimentaler Cholesterinsteatose, Beitr. Path. Anat.
   56: 379, 1913.
2. Atsumi, T., Isokane, N., Honda, Y., Matsuda, M. and Shimamoto,
   T.: Studies on atherosclerosis obliterans, tibialis anterior
   blood flow measured by Xe-133 clearance method and its clinical
   evaluation. Jap. Circ. J. 35: 1220, 1971.
3. Becker, C.G. and Murphy, G.E.: Demonstration of contractile
   protein in endothelium and cells of heart valves, endocardium,
   intima, arteriosclerotic plaques, and Aschoff bodies of rheuma-
   tic heart disease.
   Am. J. Path. 55: 1, 1969.
4. Becker, C.G. and Nachman, R.L.: Contractile proteins of
   endothelial cells, platelets and smooth muscle.
   Am. J. Path. 71: 1, 1973.
5. Bennett, H.S.: The concepts of membrane flow and membrane
   vesiculation as mechanisms for active transport and ion pum
   pumping.
   J. Biophysic. and Biochem. Cytol. 2: 99, 1956.
6. Camerini-Davalos, R.A., Ehrinereich, T., Patel, D. and
   Oppermann, W.: Nephropathy in spontaneously diabetic mice and
   its possible prevention by pyridinolcarbamate (PDC),
   in Shimamoto, T., Numano, F. and Addison, G.M. editors.
   Atherogenesis II, Excerpta Medica, 1973, p. 223.

7. Cotton, R.C., Bloor, K. and Archibald, G.:
   The effect of pyridinolcarbamate treatment on the platelet
   response to ADP in patients with peripheral atherosclerosis.
   Brit. J. Surg. 59: 313, 1972.

8. Duguid, J.B.: Thrombosis as a factor in the pathogenesis of
   aortic atherosclerosis.
   J. Path. Bact. 60: 57, 1948

9. Fukui, K.: Clinical results of pyridinolcarbamate treatment
   of hemiplegics in Kakeyu Hospital.
   Atherogenesis, Excerpta Medica, 1969, p. 239.

10. Grafnetter, D., Shimamoto, T. and Numano, F., and
    Addison, editors.
    Atherogenesis II, Excerpta Medica, 1973, p. 122.

11. Haust, M.D. and More, R.H.: Development of modern theories
    on the pathogenesis of atherosclerosis, in Wissler, R.W., and
    Geer, J.C., editors: The pathogenesis of Atherosclerosis,
    The Williams & Wilkins Co., Ltd., Baltimore, 1972, p. 1.

12. Insull, W., Jr.: Lipids in arteriosclerotic arterial tissues
    of man, in Likoff, W., Bernard, L.S. and Insull W., Jr.,
    editors: Atherosclerosis and Coronary Heart Diseases,
    Grune & Stratton, New York, 1972, p. 20.

13. Januskevichius, 2. and Bloozhas, J.
    Clinical trial of pyridinolcarbamate.
    Atherogenesis II, Excerpta Medica, 1973, p. 311.

14. Kaneko, Y.
    Plasma renin activity and prognosis of essential hypertension.
    Jap. Circ. J. 36: 995, 1972.

15. Kritchevsky, D. and Tepper, S.A.
    Influence of pyridinolcarbamate on oxidation of cholesterol
    by rat liver mitochondria.
    Arzneimittel-Forschung 21: 146, 1971.

16. Kuo, P.T.
    Plasma lipids and atherosclerosis, in ibidem, p. 8.

17. Kyusov, V.A., Belousov, Yu B., Martynov, A.I., Koroleva, S.A.,
    Zimin, V.S. and Dudaev, V.A.
    Treatment by Anginin (pyridinolcarbamate) of the coronary and
    obliterating atherosclerosis of the lower extremities.
    Cardiology 11: 39, 1972.

18. Laragh, J.H.
    Biochemical profiling and the natural history of hypertensive
    diseases: Low-renin essential hypertension, a benign condition.
    Circulation 44: 971, 1971.

19. Lofland, H.B. and Clarkson, T.B.
    The bi-directional transfer of cholesterol in normal aorta,
    fatty streaks, and atheromatous plaques.
    Proc. Soc. Exptl. Biol. Med. 133: 1, 1970.

20. Majino, G., Shea, S.M. and Leventhal, M.
    Endothelial contraction induced by histamine-type mediators.
    An electron microscopic study.
    J. Cell Biol. 42: 647, 1969.

21. Numano, F., Katsu, K., Takenobu, M., Sagara, A. and
    Shimamoto, T.
    Comparative studies on the preventive effect of pyridinol-
    carbamate and estrogen against aortic and coronary athero-
    sclerosis of cholesterol-fed rabbits. Part II:
    Histoenzymatic studies.
    Acta Path., Jap. 21: 193, 1971.
22. Resch, J.A., Okabe, N., Loewenson, R., Kimoto, K., Katsuki, S.
    and Baker, A.B.
    A comparative study of cerebral atherosclerosis in a Japanese
    and Minnesota population.
    J. Atheroscler. Res. 7: 687, 1967.
23. Robertson, A.L. and Khairallah, P.A.
    Effects of angiotensin II and some analogues on vascular
    permeability in the rabbit.
    Circ. Res. 31: 923, 1972.
24. Sano, T., Yamazaki, H. and Shimamoto, T.
    Enhancement of ADP-induced platelet aggregation by cholesterol
    and its prevention by pyridinolcarbamate.
    Thromb. Diath. haemorrh.
    In press.
25. Shimamoto, T.
    New concept on atherogenesis and treatment of
    atherosclerotic diseases with endothelial cell relaxant.
    Jap. Heart J. 13: 537, 1972.
26. Shimamoto, T.
    The relationship of edematous reaction in arteries to
    atherosclerosis and thrombosis.
    J. Atheroscler. Res. 3: 87, 1963.
27. Shimamoto, T.
    Experimental study on atherosclerosis. An attempt at its
    prevention and treatment.
    Acta Path. Jap. 19: 15, 1969.
28. Shimamoto, T., Atsumi, T., Yamashita, S., Motomiya, T.,
    Isokane, N., Ishioka, T. and Sakuma, A.
    Clinical pharmacologic evaluation of the anti-atherosclerotic
    agent, pyridinolcarbamate. A double-blind crossover trial
    in the treatment of Atherosclerosis Obliterans.
    Amer. Heart J. 79: 5, 1970.
29. Shimamoto, T., Kobayashi, M. and Numano, F.
    Infiltration of Y-globulin, fibrinogen and beta-lipoprotein
    into blood vessel wall by atherogenic stress visualized by
    immuno-fluorescence.
    Prof. Jap. Acad. 48: 336, 1972.
30. Shimamoto, T. and Numano, F.
    Preventive effect of estrogen against cholesterol-induced
    contraction of arterial endothelial cell. An electron
    microscopic observation.
    Proc. Jap. Acad. 48: 742, 1972.

31. Shimamoto, T. and Numano, F.
    Contraction and relaxation of endothelial cells covering
    atheroma and their significance.
    Prof. Jap. Acad. 49: 77, 1973.
32. Shimamoto, T. Numano, F. and Fujita, T.
    Atherosclerosis-inhibiting effect of an antibradykinin
    agent, pyridinolcarbamate.
    Amer. Heart J. 71: 216, 1966.
33. Shimamoto, T. and Sunaga, T.
    Contraction of endothelial cells as a key mechanism in
    atherogenesis.
    Prof. Jap. Acad. 48: 633, 1972.
34. Shimamoto, T. and Sunaga, T.
    The contraction and blebbing of endothelial cells
    accompanied by acute infiltration of plasma substances
    into the vessel wall and their prevention, in Shimamoto, T.,
    Numano, F. and Addison, G.M., editor.
    Atherogenesis II, Excerpta, Medica, 1973, p.3.
35. Shimamoto, T. and Yamazaki, H.
    Bradykinin-antagonistic anti-inflammatory substance B23
    in treatment of angina pectoris.
    Proc. 3rd Asian-Pacific Cong. Cardiology, Kyoto, 1964, p. 748.
36. Shkhvatsabaya, I.K.
    Anginin in the treatment of patients with chronic
    coronary insufficiency.
    Atherogenesis II, Excerpta Medica, 1973, p. 347.
37. Stamler, J., Berkson, D.N. and Lindberg, H.A.
    Risk factors: Their role in the etiology and pathogenesis
    of the atherosclerotic diseases, in Wissler, R.W. and
    Geer, J.C., editors.
    The Pathogenesis of Atherosclerosis, The Williams & Wilkins
    Co., Ltd., Baltimore, 1972, p. 41.
38. Wu, C.C., Huang, T.S. and Hsu, C.J.
    Prevention of experimental atherosclerosis with
    pyridinolcarbamate.
    Amer. Heart J. 77: 657, 1969.
39. Yamamura, T.
    Inhibitory effects of pyridinolcarbamate in angiolathyrism
    and osteolathyrism, in Shimamoto, T. and Numano, F., editors.
    Atherogenesis, Excerpta Medica, 1969, p. 29.
40. Yamazaki, H., Takahashi, T. and Shimamoto, T.
    Inhibitory action of acetylsalicilic acid, pyridinolcarbamate
    and its derivative on human platelet aggregation.
    Blood & Vessel 3: 1377, 1972.
41. Yamazawa, S., Shimamoto, T., Hidaka, H. and Mohri, K.
    The search for anti-atherosclerotic agents. Histological
    and chemical analysis of the preventive effect of estrogen,
    progesterone and pyridinolcarbamate on experimentally induced
    atherosclerosis.
    Atherogenesis II, Excerpta Medica, 1973, p. 98.

THE EFFECTS OF LIPIDS AND FATTY ACIDS ON BLOOD COAGULATION

AND PLATELETS IN RELATION TO THROMBOSIS

E.F. LÜSCHER

Theodor Kocher Institute, University of Berne

Thrombosis is an often encountered consequence of atherosclerotic alterations of the vessel wall, and there can be no doubt that in its genesis, blood platelets play a predominant role (cf.55). Platelets in turn are of considerable interest as the model of a metabolically active, contractile cell, capable of reacting to a variety of external stimuli. In the course of their "activation", they display a series of morphological and biochemical alterations, in the course of which they aggregate and acquire procoagulant properties. It is of particular interest that lipids and fatty acids are known to interact with platelets and with the blood clotting system, and this again justifies the inclusion of a chapter on thrombosis in this series of articles on diet and atherosclerosis.

1. Lipids and blood coagulation - In Fig. 1 is shown a simplified scheme of blood coagulation, subdivided into the extrinsic and intrinsic pathways of prothrombin activation.

The extrinsic pathway is based on the availability of tissue thromboplastin, a phospholipoprotein procoagulant found in most tissue cells, as well as in erythrocytes and leukocytes. It is made available whenever such cells are injured by a variety of means. Small amounts of tissue thromboplastin are capable of activating prothrombin by the extrinsic pathway within seconds. As a consequence, its intravascular application may lead to immediate thrombin formation and vascular occlusion.

In the intrinsic system, phospholipid again is required. There are two steps involved: the first involving the activation of factor X, the second of prothrombin. In whole blood this phospholipid procoagulant is provided by the blood platelets, because they alone are capable of making it available in the course of the activation of the clotting system. Platelet phospholipoprotein

107

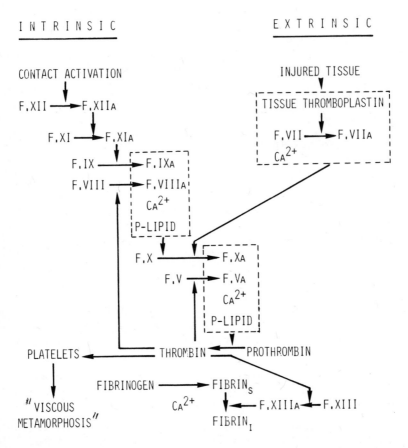

Fig. 1. Schematic representation of the blood clotting process

The term "viscous metamorphosis" is meant to designate the total of the changes accompanying irreversible aggregation under the influence of thrombin, i.e. release reaction, activation of the contractile system, and availability of phospholipid procoabulant (PF 3).

(or phospholipids isolated from it), often termed platelet factor 3 (PF 3), is not a rate-determining factor in prothrombin activation. It can be applied intravascularly without any dramatic effect. This becomes understandable in view of the fact that its activity depends on a time consuming reaction and, first of all, on the presence, at the same time, of activated clotting factors. According to Fig. 1, these are in particular the activated forms of factors XI (XIa) and IX (IXa). In vitro, the activation of factor XI is mainly brought about by factor XIIa (activated Hageman-factor). Only recently has been demonstrated that PF3-lipoprotein (but not the phospholipid alone) is also capable of activating directly factor XI (57).

Tissue thromboplastin as well as PF3 are membrane constituents which differ mainly in their portein moiety. Circulating platelets display no procoagulant activity, this although undoubtedly a large part of their external surface is composed of phospholipids. It is only in the course of their "activation", that their surface becomes active in the clotting process. Zwaal, Roelofsen and Colley (61) have recently described that the erythrocyte membrane is character- ized by a strict orientation of the phospholipids within the lipid bilayer: on the outside are found mostly lecithin and sphingomyelin, whereas phosphatidylethanolamine and phosphatidylserine are located mainly on the inside. This is of special interest, because only the latter two phosphatides are active in blood coagulation. Provided similar conditions are realized in the platelet membrane, this might mean that the availability of PF3 reflects a dramatic, inside-out re- arrangement of the structural elements of the plasma membrane.

Damaged cells, membrane fragments, and the activator complexes of the intrinsic system are as a rule rapidly eliminated from cir- culation. It thus seems unlikely that phospholipid procoagulants will accumulate in circulation. If they do, the effect should con- sist in a general activation of the clotting system, provided the contact factors, in particular factor XIa, are also present in ade- quate amounts. Increased plasma levels of "cephalins" have never- theless been described with less dramatic results in patients with hyperlipemia and with coronary heart disease (37).

Free fatty acids may directly activate the contact factors (17, 47) and thus also contribute to an activated state of the clotting system. However, as will be discussed later, their effect on the platelets is much more pronounced, and in turn may lead to platelet- mediated contact activation.

According to Egeberg (10), factor XI is found activated after a fat-rich meal, whereas other authors, even after feeding up to 118 g of a mixture of saturated and unsaturated fats find no eviden- ce whatsoever for an activation of the blood clotting system (31). It is obvious that the methodology of such experiments is decisive for their outcome.

2. <u>The activation of the platelets</u> - The inert, circulating platelet can undergo a series of far-reading alterations in the course of which it becomes capable of aggregation and of the participation in blood coagulation.

The inducers of these alterations range from certain proteolytic enzymes, in particular thrombin, to large molecules such as collagen, immune complexes, zymosan (alpha 41) and cationic polymers (alpha 28), and, finally, low molecular weight compounds such as adenosine-5-diphosphate (ADP), adrenaline, vasopressin, and serotonin. This wide variety of materials, all of them capable of eliciting the same result, suggests that upon quite different stimuli of the plasma membrane, the same sequence of events is triggered off. These events can be subdivided by several criteria in different phases:

- A "rapid shape change", in the course of which the disk-shaped platelet is transformed, within seconds, into an irregular sphere.

- A primary aggregation, which may be spontaneously reversible, provided a given threshold concentration of the inducing agent is not exceeded.

- Irreversible or second phase aggregation with higher than threshold concentrations of inducer. In its course, tightly packed platelet masses are formed. These represent the building material of a functional "hemostatic plug" closing an injured blood vessel, or of the "white thrombus" occluding an artery at the site of injured endothelium.

- A release reaction, which invariably accompanies irreversible aggregation. This reaction is defined as a fast, specific process, terminated within the first minute after stimulation of the platelet by an adequately high concentration of any of the above mentioned inducing agents. In its course the contents of specific storage organelles (socalled dense bodies and alpha-granules) are emptied to the outside of the cell (alpha 18). This obviously must involve the fusion of two membrane systems, i.e. the plasma membrane and the organelle membrane(s). Released are from human platelets:Serotonin, small amounts of adrenaline, adenine nucleotides including considerable amounts of ADP, a heparin-neutralizing factor, fibrinogen, Ca^{2+} and K^+-ions, to mention only the most important components.

It is particularly noteworthy that among the released materials are found several (ADP, adrenaline, serotonin) which in turn are capable of eliciting by themselves the release reaction. ADP, the most important inducer, depends for its activity on the presence of fibrinogen and Ca^{2+}-ions; both are also released, thus establishing a self-contained system capable of the further propagation of irreversible aggregation independent of the external medium.

- The availability of procoagulant PF3, which follows with some delay the release reaction proper.

- The activation of the contractile system of the platelet. Up to 15% of the platelet's protein are accounted for by an actomyosin-like, contractile protein, termed thrombosthenin, which depends for its activation on Ca^{2+}-ions and a regulatory system closely related to the one of muscle (27). It is thought that contractile activity is essential for the formation, in the case of arterial thrombosis, of a tight platelet aggregate, capable of withstanding the eroding forces of arterial circulation.

It thus is evident that many stimuli may trigger off this sequence of events. It is particularly noteworthy that, according to several authors, lipids and fatty acids also belong to the series of inducing agents and, under certain circumstances, must be looked upon as potentially thrombogenic materials.

In the past years a considerable literature has accumulated on this subject. There is general agreement that free fatty acids exert a direct influence on blood platelets, be it in vitro, or under in vivo conditions. This effect is most pronounced with longchain, saturated comounds (1,16,17,22,47,60): they give rise to platelet alterations culminating in the release reaction; further aggregation then ensues via the ADP-mechanism (14). Interestingly enough, the aggregation-inducing effect of Na-stearate was considerably less pronounced when the platelets were suspended in a factor XII-deficient plasma (17). This might mean that the final effect is due to a superposition of a direct effect, and of the local activation of the clotting system via the contact factors. This might also explain, why the pre-treatment of rats with saturated fatty acids (and cholesterol) leads to the death by thrombosis of the animals upon injection of ADP (36).

The addition of lipid emulsions to platelets leads to the uptake of lipid particles by phagocytosis (19,32,40,45). In most cases, this is linked to membrane impairment (32,40); however, the absence of such alterations 22 hours after the infusion of sojbean lipids has been reported recently (19). Here again, the experimental procedures used, appear decisive for the final outcome.

Hyperlipemia produced by fat feeding seems not to exert a pronounced, direct effect on platelets (9); on the other hand, there is general agreement that this conditions is an important contributory factor towards aggregation and thrombus formation (5,42). According to Farbiszewski et al. (11) it is mainly the beta-lipoprotein fraction which is responsible for this effect; in the hands of these authors, the alpha-lipoproteins were inactive, and chylomicra showed an effect only at high concentrations. A most interesting possible explanation for the special role of low density lipoprotein (LDL) on platelets has been brought forward by Bolton, Hampton and Mitchell (3). According to these authors, the labilizing effect of the platelet membrane (which is discernible by an altered surface charge) is due to the appearance of lysolecithin, which is formed from LDL and a labile phospholipase, most likely of platelet origin. This phospholipase is unable to react with high density lipoproteins.

Finally it should be noted that induced allimentary hyperlipemia also favours the adhesion of platelets in in vitro and in vivo systems (12,33,35).

The hope that highly unsaturated fatty acids, in particular linolenic acid may be of prophylactic value in hypercholesterolemia-linked coronary heart disease (via the depression of enhanced platelet adhesivity due to increased von Willebrand-factor activities [2,38]) unfortunately has been dispelled by extensive clinical trial (34,39).

3. Fatty acid metabolism of platelets and prostaglandins -

Fatty acids are rapidly taken up by platelet in the presence of albumin. They are then metabolized or incorporated, primarily into lecithin, but in other lipids as well (6,8,51).

The fact that platelets are capable of metabolizing fatty acids, has recently promoted an increasing number of studies on the possible relationship of the effects of fatty acids to prostaglandins (PG). PGE_1 is for some time known as one of the most powerful inhibitors of platelet aggregation and of the release reaction (15,23,24,25).

However, PGE_1 is neither contained in, nor synthesized by the platelets. On the other hand, PGE_2 is capable of supporting ADP-induced platelet aggregation (7,46), and it is at the same time a platelet constituent, synthesized from arachidonic acid (21,44). This synthesis is particularly pronounced in the course of aggregation (48,49). It has recently been suggested that it is not PGE_2 which is responsible for the observed potentiating effect on platelet aggregation, but another, labile product, most likely of the same, PGE_2-synthesizing enzyme system (58).

The question then arises, how the prostaglandins influence platelet activity. For PGE_1 it is established that it acts by activating adenyl cyclase (alpha 55,56) and it has been shown recently that, conversely, PGE_2 inhibits this enzyme (43). Cyclic 3',5'-adenosine monophosphate (cAMP) is known to exert a dominant control function on platelet activity alpha 27): high levels of the nucleotide tend to stabilize it in the inert form, lowered levels favour aggregation, release and contractility. It is of special interest that acetyl salicylic acid, a potent inhibitor of second phase platelet aggregation, is also a blocker of the synthesis of PGE_2 and PGF_{2alpha} in platelets which are triggered into

activity by thrombin (48,59). Accordingly, the preincubation of
platelets with arachidonic acid (in the presence of adequate reducing agents) prevents the inhibitory effect of acetyl salicylic acid
on aggregation (26).

Fatty acids therefore, functioning as the precursor molecules
of the prostaglandins, in particular PGE_2, may well play a most
important role in the control of platelet activities in relation
to their aggregation and to thrombosis.

4.   Thrombus formation and the vascular wall - There is general agreement that arterial thrombosis starts out from an endothelial lesion to which platelets adhere, and, by subsequent aggregation and release of aggregation-inducers, give raise to an
obstructing "white thrombus", followed later-on by a "red thrombus"
consisting of fibrin and trapped blood cells (alpha 55). Thus, in
the sequence of events, the first step consists in the adhesion of
the circulating platelets to the injured endo-thelium. Endothelial
cells themselves are not capable of trapping platelets. It seems
a prerequisit for platelet adhesion that the subendothelial lining
becomes accessible. Several structures to which platelets adhere
have been defined: the basement membrane, collagen, and the socalled subendothelial fibrils (20,52,54, cf. also 50). Apparently,
this implies rather gross damage to the endothelium, e.g. a ruptured atherosclerotic plaque. However, it has been shown that platelets will also adhere to miniature gaps between endothelial cells
(53), and the question arises, whether not the movement due to the
well established contractile properties of these cells (13,29) is
in some instances sufficient for platelet adhesion. There is also
increasing eveidence that endothelial cells may be dislodged from
their positions by a variety of agents, such as endotoxin (30) or
even thrombin (4). It seems of interest to await further experiments, devised to demonstrate what the prerequisits for platelet
adhesion to the altered vascular endothelium really are. There
can be little doubt that new and interesting results are to be expected from such an approach which must be based on a much more
dynamic picture of the endothelial cell, which is, like the platelet, a contractile element, vulnerable to a variety of external stimuli. The fact that both cells are affected directly or indirectly
by lipids and fatty acids, may turn out to be of particular interest in the context of the present topic.

REFERENCES

1. Ardlie, N.G., Kinlough, R.L., Glew, G. and Schwartz, C.J.:
   Fatty acids and in vitro platelet aggregation.
   Aust. J. Exp. Biol. Med. Sci. 44: 105, 1966.
2. Böhles, E., Bauke, J., Harmuth, E. and Breddin, K.:
   Untersuchungen über die Agglutination der Blutplättchen nach
   Zufuhr verschiedener Nahrungsfette.
   Klin. Wschr. 43: 555, 1965.
3. Bolton, C.H., Hampton, J.R. and Mitchell, J.R.A.:
   Nature of the transferable factor which causes abnormal
   platelet behaviour in vascular disease.
   Lancet II: 1101, 1967.
4. Booyse, F.M., Shepro, D., Rosenthal, M., McDonald, R.I.:
   Properties of cultured endothelial cells.
   Ser. Haemat. 6
   In press
5. Born, G.V.R. and Philp, R.B.:
   Effects of adenosine analogues and of heparin on platelet
   thrombi in non-lipaemic and lipaemic rats.
   Brit. J. Exper. Pathol. 46: 569, 1965.
6. Cohen, P., Derksen, A. and van den Bosch, H.:
   Pathways of fatty acid metabolism in human platelets.
   J. Clin. Invest. 49: 128, 1970.
7. Creveld van, S. and Pascha, C.N.:
   Abnormality in the aggregation of blood platelets in various
   morbid conditions and the influence of prostaglandins upon
   this abnormality.
   Thrombos. Diathes. Haemorrh. 20: 180, 1968.
8. Deykind, D. and Desser, R.K.:
   The incorporation of acetate and palmitate into lipids
   by human platelets.
   J. Clin. Invest. 47: 1590, 1968.
9. Dubber, A.H.C., Rifkind, B., Gale, M., McNicol, G.P. and
   Douglas, A.S.:
   Effect of fat feeding on fibrinolysisn stypven time and
   platelet aggregation.
   J. Atheroscler. Res. 7: 225, 1967.
10. Egeberg, O.: Blood Factor XI after fat-rich meals.
    Thrombos. Diathes. Haemorrh. 15: 390, 1966.
11. Farbiszewski, R., Skrzydlewski, Z. and Worowski, K.:
    The effect of lipoprotein fractions on adhesiveness and
    aggregation of blood platelets.
    Thrombos. Diathes. Haemorrh. 21: 89, 1969.
12. Frost, H.: Zur Pathogenese obliterierender Arterienprozesse
    bei Hypercholesterinämie.
    Thrombos. Diathes. Haemorrh. 22: 351, 1969.
13. Giacomelli, F., Wiener, J. and Spiro, D.:
    Cross-striated arrays of filaments in endothelium.
    J. Cell Biol. 45: 188, 1970.

14. Haslam, R.J.: Role of adenosine diphosphate in the aggregation
    of human blood platelets by thrombin and by fatty acids.
    Nature, Lond. 202: 765, 1964.
15. Hissen, W., Fleming, J.S., Bierwagen, M.E. and Pindell M.H.:
    Effect of prostaglandin PGE$_1$ on platelet aggregation in vitro
    and in hemorrhagic shock.
    Microvascular Res. 1: 374, 1969.
16. Hoak, J.C.: Structure of thrombi produced by the injection
    of fatty acids.
    Brit. J. Exper. Pathol. 45: 44, 1964.
17. Hoak, J.C., Warner, E.D. and Connor, W.E.:
    Platelets, fatty acids and thrombosis.
    Circulat. Res. 20: 11, 1967.
18. Holmsen, H., Day, H.J. and Stormorken, H.:
    The blood platelet release reaction.
    Scand. J. Haemat., Suppl. 2, 1969.
19. Hovig, T. and Grøttum, K.A.: Lipid infusions in man -
    Ultrastructural studies on blood platelet uptake of
    fat particles.
    Thrombos. Diathes. Haemorrh. 29, 450, 1973.
20. Hugues, J. and Mahieu, P.: Platelet aggregation induced by
    basement membranes.
    Thrombos. Diathes. Haemorrh. 24: 395, 1970.
21. Ingerman, C., Smith, J.B., Kocsis, J.J. and Silver, M.J.:
    Arachidonic acid induces platelet aggregation and
    platelet prostaglandin formation.
    Fed. Proc. 32: 219, 1973.
22. Kerr, J.W., Pirrie, R. and Bronte-Stewart, B.:
    Platelet aggregation by phospholipids and free fatty acids.
    Lancet I: 1296, 1965.
23. Kinlough-Rathbone, R.L., Packham, M.A. and Mustard, J.F.:
    The effect of prostaglandin E$_1$ on platelet function in vitro
    and in vivo.
    Brit. J. Haemat. 19: 559, 1970.
24. Kloeze, J.: Prostaglandins and platelet aggregation in vivo.
    II. Influence of PGE$_{1alpha}$ on platelet thrombus formation
    induced by an electric stimulus in veins on the rat brain
    surface.
    Thrombos. Diathes. Haemorrh. 23: 293, 1970.
25. Kloeze, J. and Hornstra, G.: Effects of prostaglandin on
    platelet aggregation and experimental thrombosis in
    Platelet Aggregation, J. Caen, ed.;
    Masson, Paris, p. 165-172, 1971.
26. Leonardi, R.G., Alexander, B. and White, F.:
    Prevention of the inhibitory effect of aspirin on platelet
    aggregation.
    Fed. Proc. 31: 248, 1972.

27. Lüscher, E.F. and Bettex-Galland, M.:
    Thrombosthenin, the contractile protein of blood platelets.
    New facts and problems.
    Path. Biol. 20, suppl. 89-101, 1972.
28. Lüscher, E.F., Pfueller, S.L. and Massini, P.:
    Platelet aggregation by large molecules.
    Ser. Haemat. 6: 382, 1973.
29. Majno, G., Shea, S.M. and Leventhal, M.:
    Endothelial contraction as a mechanism of action of
    histamine-type mediators. An electro-microscopic study.
    J. Cell Biol. 42: 647, 1969.
30. McGrath, J.M. and Stewart, G.J.:
    The effects of endotoxin on vascular endothelium.
    J. Exper. Med. 129: 833, 1969.
31. Meuwissen, O.J.A.Th., Hart, H. Ch. and van Hemal-Rupert, M.S.E.:
    The influence of fats on blood coagulation and fibrinolysis.
    Thrombos. Diathes. Haemorrh. 19: 267, 1968.
32. Morgenstern, E., Pfleiderer, Th., Zebisch, P. and Weber, E.:
    Ueber die Wirkung von Lipidemulsionen auf Blutplättchen.
    II. Licht- und elektronenmikroskopische Studien.
    Thrombos. Diathes. Haemorrh. 22: 525, 1969.
33. Mustard, J.F., Rowsell, H.C., Murphy, E.A. and Downie, H.G.:
    Diet and thrombus formation; quantitative studies using an
    extracorporeal circulation in pigs.
    J. Clin. Invest. 42: 1783, 1963.
34. Natvig, H., Borchgrevink, C.F., Dedichen, J., Owren, P.A.,
    Schløtz, E.H. and Westlund, K.: A controlled trial of the
    effect of linolenic acid on incidence of coronary heart
    disease.
    Scand. J. Clin. Lab. Invest. 22: suppl. 105, 1968.
35. Nordöy, A.: The influence of saturated fat, cholesterol,
    cern oil and linseed oil on the ADP-induced platelet
    adhesiveness in the rat.
    Thrombos. Diathes. Haemorrh. 13: 543, 1965.
36. Nordöy, A. and Chandler, A.B.:
    The influence of dietary fats on the adenosine diphosphate
    induced platelet thrombosis in the rat.
    Scand. J. Haemat. 1: 202, 1964.
37. Nothman, M.M. and Proger, S.:
    Cephalins in the blood. Patients with coronary heart
    disease and patients with hyperlipemia.
    J.A.M.A. 179: 40, 1962.
38. Owren, P.A.: Coronary thrombosis. Its mechanism and possible
    prevention by linolenic acid.
    Ann. Intern. Med. 63: 167, 1965.
39. Owren, P.A., Hellem, A. and Ødegaard, A.:
    Linolenic acid and platelet adhesiveness.
    Lancet II, 849, 1965.

40. Pfleiderer, TH., Morgenstern, E. and Weber, E.:
    Ueber die Wirkung von Lipidemulsionen auf Blutplättchen.
    I. Zunahme der Plättchenaggregation unter dem Einfluss
    verschiedener Libidemulsionen in vitro.
    Thrombos. Diathes. Haemorrh. 22: 513, 1969.
41. Pfueller, S.L. and Lüscher, E.F.:
    Studies on the mechanism of the human platelet release
    reaction induced by immunological stimuli.
    II. The effects of zymosan.
    J. Immunol.
    In press.
42. Renzenbrink, J., Holzknecht, F. and Braunsteiner, H.:
    Erhöhte Aggregation der Thrombocyten bei essentieller
    Hyperlipämie.
    Acta Haemat. 38, 95, 1967.
43. Salzman, E.W., Kensler, E.W. and Levine, L.:
    Cyclic 3', 5'-adenosine monophosphate in human blood platelets.
    IV. Regulatory role of cyclic AMP in platelet function. In:
    Platelets and their role in hemostasis.
    Ann. N.Y. Acad. Sci., 201: 61, 1972.
44. Schoene, N.W., Dutky, R.C. and Iacono, J.M.:
    Biosynthesis of prostaglandin E_2 in human blood platelets
    from 1-^{14}C-Arachidonic acid.
    Circulation 46: II : 32, 1972.
45. Schulz, H. and Wedell, J.:
    Elektronenmikroskopische Untersuchungen zur Frage der
    Fettphagocytose und des Fett-transportes durch Thrombocyten.
    Klin. Wschr. 40: 1114, 1962.
46. Shio, H. and Ramwell, P.:
    Effect of prostaglandin E_2 and aspirin on the secondary
    aggregation of human platelets.
    Nature New Biology 236: 45, 1972.
47. Shore, P.A. and Alpers, H.S.:
    Platelet damage induced in plasma by certain fatty acids.
    Nature, Lond., 200: 1331, 1963.
48. Smith, J.B. and Willis, A.L.:
    Aspirin selectively inhibits prostaglandin production
    in human platelets.
    Nature New Biology 231: 235, 1971.
49. Smith, J.G., Ingerman, C., Kocsis, J.J. and Silver, M.J.:
    Formation of prostaglandins during the aggregation of human
    blood platelets.
    J. Clin. Invest. 52: 965, 1973.
50. Spaet, T.H. and Stemerman, M.B.:
    Platelet adhesion.
    Ann. N.Y. Acad. Sci. 201: 13, 1972.
51. Spector, A.A., Hoak, J.C., Warner, E.D. and Fry, G.L.:
    Utilization of long-chain free fatty acids by human platelets.
    J. Clin. Invest. 49: 1489, 1970.

52. Stemerman, M.B., Baumgartner, H.R. and Spaet, T.H.
    The subendothelial microfibril and platelet adhesion.
    Lab. Invest. 24: 179, 1971.
53. Trancer, J.P. and Baumgartner, H.R.
    Filling gaps in the vascular endothelium with
    blood platelets.
    Nature 216: 1126, 1967.
54. T'sao, C.H. and Glasgov, S.: Platelet adhesion to subendothelial
    components in experimental aortic injury. Role of fine fibrils
    and basement memebrane.
    Brit. J. Exper. Path. 51: 423, 1970.
55. Vermylen, J., de Gaetano, G. and Verstraete, M.
    Platelets and thrombosis. In: Recent Advances in Thrombosis.
    L. Poller, ed. (Churchill, Livingstone, London 1973) p. 113-150.
56. Vigdahl, R.L., Marquis, N.R. and Tavormina, P.A.
    Platelet aggregation. II. Adenyl cyclase, prostaglandin E_1
    and calcium.
    Biochem. Biophys. Res. Comm. 37: 409, 1969.
57. Walsh, P.N.
    Platelet coagulant activities: evidence for
    multiple, different function of platelets in intrinsic
    coagulation.
    Ser. Haemat. 6: 1973.
    In press.
58. Willis, A.L.
    An enzymatic mechanism for the anti-thrombotic and
    anti-hemostatic actions of aspirin.
    Science
    In press.
59. Willis, A.L. and Kuhn, D.C.
    A new potential mediator of arterial thrombosis whose
    biosynthesis is inhibited by aspirin.
    Prostaglandins 4: 127, 1973.
60. Zbinden, G.
    Lauric acid-induced thrombocytopenia and
    thrombosis in rabbits.
    Thrombos. Diathes. Haemorrh. 18: 57, 1967.
61. Zwaal, R.A., Roelofsen, B. and Colley, C.M.
    Localization of red cell membrane constituents.
    Biochim. Biophys. Acta 300: 159, 1973.

DIAGNOSTIC METHODS FOR THE STUDY OF HUMAN ATHEROSCLEROSIS

D. H. BLANKENHORN, M.D.

University of Southern California

ATHEROSCLEROSIS DIAGNOSIS AND ATHEROMA ASSESSMENT

Almost all individuals over 30 years of age in Western Europe and the United States are known to have some degree of atherosclerosis. Myocardial infarction, angina pectoris, peripheral vascular insufficiency, and cerebral ischemia are sequelae of atherosclerosis. It is generally correct to assume that any individual manifesting these sequelae has atherosclerosis and this is the rationale underlying most diagnostic procedures. For example, occurrence of myocardial infarction or its prodromata leads to the diagnosis of coronary atherosclerosis. This is the conventional approach to ATHEROSCLEROSIS DIAGNOSIS.

End organ damage might be avoided in many cases if we could detect and treat atheromatous lesions in their early stages. Experiments have provided substantial evidence that atheromatous lesions can be made to regress in animals (1). If means were available to ascertain whether atheromas were regressing or becoming more severe in man, choice of drugs or diet for therapy could be based on observation of their effectiveness for each individual patient. The information required is knowledge of how many plaques exist in a given vessel and whether they are early lesions, raised lesions, or lesions complicated by ulceration, calcification, or hemorrhage. Two techniques for ATHEROMA ASSESSMENT can now obtain a part of the information and have potential for serial use as therapy monitors. Table I presents various methods now available for ATHEROSCLEROSIS DIAGNOSIS and ATHEROMA ASSESSMENT.

Table I.   ATHEROSCLEROSIS DIAGNOSIS

A.   Flow Dependent
    1. Plethysmography
    2. Segmental pulse velocity determination
    3. Phonoangiography
    4. Any of the above before and after reactive hyperemia

B.   Ischemia Detection
    1. Cardiac
        EKG
        VCG
        With or without exercise testing
    2. Peripheral skin temperature measurement
    3. Cerebral thermography

C.   Angiography with Conventional Clinical Goals

ATHEROMA ASSESSMENT

A.   Roentgenography for Vascular Calcification

B.   Angiography with Quantitative Measurement for
      Image Interpretation

ATHEROSCLEROSIS DIAGNOSIS

    Subdivision of these methods into the classes – flow depend-
ent and ischemia detection – is arbitrary because significant reduction of blood flow leads to ischemia. In the cerebral circulation where reduced blood flow leads to prompt ischemic damage
methods measuring the two phenomenon are virtually indistinguish-
able. In peripheral circulation where reduced blood flow can be
tolerated for prolonged periods methods measuring the two phenomena can be quite different. The cardiac circulation lies between
cerebral and peripheral in the speed with which flow reduction
leads to ischemia. Most of the discussion which follows will deal
with the peripheral and cardiac circulatory beds.

Flow Dependent

Plethysmography - This is applied to the peripheral circulation and is a measurement of blood flow by calculating changes in volume of an extremity. Venous outflow is occluded and subsequent change in leg volume is an indication of the amount of arterial blood passing into the occluded area. The effect of treatment has been studied in patients with hyperlipoproteinemia by plethysmographic measurement of peak reactive hyperemia blood flow (2). The results are noteworthy because the direct effect of therapy for hyperlipoproteinemia on a measurable blood vessel response was demonstrated.

Segmental pulse velocity determinations - Segmental pulse velocity determination has a long history, it was one of the earliest methods proposed for atheroma assessment. The current consensus is that the elastic properties of blood vessel wall, not atherosclerosis, are the major determinant of pulse wave velocity (3,4). The elasticity of blood vessel walls diminishes with age and pulse velocity increases whether or not ahterosclerosis also occurs.

Phonoangiography - This is detection and recording of vascular bruits or murmurs (5). Lesions which narrow the vessel lumen by 50 to 70% produce sufficient intra-vascular turbulence so that recordable murmurs occur. This allows estimation of the parameters of arterial diameter, flow velocity, and wall pressure fluctuations. It is a screening tool for serial measurements to evaluate changes induced by therapy. Any factor altering cardiac output or the viscosity of blood, for example anemia, can introduce significant error.

Any of the above before and after reactive hyperemia - In the presence of occlusive arterial disease exercise produces a transient decrease (rather than the normal increase) in blood pressure in the ankle and foot. When measurements are made applying a combination of the technique above with reactive hyperemia, there is more sensitivity for discernment of small lesions. The specificity of the test is not increased however. For example, the effect of anemia altering vascular bruits would not be eliminated by combining exercise with phonoangiography.

Ischemia Detection

Cardiac - EKG and VCG - The electrocardiogram and the vectorcardiogram are conventionally used for study of cardiac ischemia. They both can be employed with or without preliminary exercise.

Peripheral skin temperature measurement - Skin temperature is useful for detecting arterial insufficiency. The most common means is to apply small thermistors at various levels on the extremities. Blood skin temperature will be lower where blood flow is reduced. The method requires careful control of ambient temperature. The

principles of peripheral ischemia detection by thermal methods can
also be applied to cerebral circulation.

Angiography with Conventional Clinical Goals

These goals are to outline obstructive lesions, fill collateral
circulation, and evaluate the capacity of run off vessels. Conventional angiography fulfills these goals, but yields little information regarding plaque prevalence or characteristics. It is generally assumed that the obstruction visualized by conventional angiograms are due to atherosclerosis, although thrombi occasionally
mimic atherosclerotic obstruction.

ATHEROMA ASSESSMENT

Roentgenography for Vascular Calcification

The atheromatous plaque develops plate-like areas of calcium
which have a characteristic roentgenographic appearance clearly
distinguishable from non-atherosclerotic calcification which occurs
in peripheral, carotid, and cerebral vessels. In the coronary artery visualization of calcification is pathognomonic for atherosclerosis; no other forms of vascular calcification occur (6).
The major limitation to the use of roentgenography for atherosclerotic calcification as an atheroma assessment method is that calcium
occurs principally in late lesions. Atheromatous calcification is
a terminal process; a deposit in dead or dying tissue.

Angiography with Quantitative Measurement
for Image Interpretation

There is information in angiograms which can lead to assessment of atheroma size and configuration. For this an image dissector linked to a digital computer is used to make pultiple measurements of vessel edge irregularity and lumen variation. During this
process, densities on the radiographic film are converted to digital data, processed by computer, and then converted back to a picture. First, the film is back lighted and viewed with the computer
controlled image dissector. This device scans the image line by
line measuring the transmitted light at 50 micron intervals and
converts the measurement into digital form which it relays to the
computer. As the picture is scanned a television display indicates
the area under study. The computer next processes digital data
from the input image using algorithms described below and generates
new data to be used for an output picture. Output pictures are
created with a device which generates a spot of light on the face
of a cathode ray tube moving in raster light sweeps across an un-
exposed film. The intensity of the light is controlled by the digital data for the output picture. In this way a reproduction of

the original angiogram is generated which indicates information added or changed by the computer.

Computer processing of image data begins with vessel edge location. For this, lines are scanned perpendicular to the vessel and each of these lines is examined left to right to see where film density shows greatest rate of change. The point at which greatest positive change (maximum slope) is found is designated as the left edge and the point at which the greatest negative change (minimum slope) is found is designated the right edge. Edge irregularity is computed separately for left and right edges by comparing the fit of curves generated from running averages.

Measurement of luminal variation is another means of assessment of atheromas. Once vessel edges on each scan line across the vessel are known, vessel midline is indicated by putting a smooth curve through all midpoints. Next, lumen edge is estimated by broadening the midline horizontally until it includes 95% of the originally detected edge points. The relative amount of disease in any portion of the vessel is proportional to the difference between the detected edges and the estimated lumen.

We have applied these methods to measurement of angiograms performed in patients who attend our clinic for hyperlipoproteinemia (7). We have compared these measurements to results of a series of postmortem examinations (8,9). The measurements obtained postmortem and those found in vivo indicate the technique has practical clinical application.

REFERENCES

1. Armstrong, M.L., Warner, E.D. and Connor, W.E.
   Regression of coronary atheromatosis in Rhesus monkeys.
   Circ. Res. 27: 59, 1970.
2. Zelis, R., Mason, D.T., Braunwald, E. and Levy, R.I.
   Effects of hyperlipoproteinemia and their treatment
   on the peripheral circulation.
   J. Clin. Invest. 49: 1007, 1970.
3. Hyman, C., Winsor, T., Fischer, E.K. and Sibley, A.E.
   Influence of vascular disease on the rate of transmission of
   various pure frequency components of the arterial pulse wave.
   Proc. IV International Congress of Angiology 756, 1961.
4. Hallock, P. and Benson, I.C.
   Studies on the elastic properties of human isolated aorta.
   J. Clin. Invest. 16: 595, 1937.
5. Lees, R.W. and Dewey, C.F. Jr.
   Phonoangiography: A new noninvasive diagnostic method for
   studying arterial disease.
   Proc. National Acad. Sci. 67: 935, 1970.

6. Blankenhorn, D.H.
   Coronary arterial calcification. A review.
   Am. J. Med. Sci. 242: 41, 1961.
7. Blankenhorn, D.H., Barndt, R. Jr., Crawford, D.W.,
   Selzer, R.H. and Beckenbach, E.S.
   Prevalence and distribution of femoral atheromas in human
   hyperlipoproteinemia, Types II and IV.
   Proc. Third International Symposium on Atherosclerosis, 1973.
   In press.
8. Crawford, D.W., Beckenbach, E.S., Blankenhorn, D.H.,
   Selzer, R.H. and Brooks, S.H.
   Grading of coronary atherosclerosis: Comparison of a modified
   IAP visual grading method and a new quantitative angiographic
   technique.
   Atherosclerosis 19: 231, 1974.
9. Blankenhorn, D.H., Brooks, S.H., Selzer, R.H.,
   Crawford, D.W. and Chin, H.P.
   Assessment of atherosclerosis from angiographic images.
   Proc. Soc. Exp. Biol. & Med.
   In press.

This work was supported by USPHS grants HL 14138 and RR-43.

DIET-RELATED RISK FACTORS FOR HUMAN ATHEROSCLEROSIS:

HYPERLIPIDEMIA, HYPERTENSION, HYPERGLYCEMIA -- CURRENT STATUS

J. STAMLER, M.D.

Professor and Chairman and Harry W. Dingman
Professor of Cardiology
Northwestern University The Medical School

A vast literature exists on the relationship between nutrition, nutrition-related risk factors, and the contemporary epidemic of atherosclerotic disease - especially coronary heart disease - in the industrialized countries (1-4). At the onset in this survey, it is worth emphasizing a point often forgotten due to the understandable preoccupation of atherosclerosis researchers with composition (quality) of the diet - especially lipid composition as it affects serum cholesterol: Nutrition is involved in the etiology of atherosclerotic disease not only via composition of the diet, especially saturated fat and cholesterol intake and the influence of these on serum cholesterol. Quantity is also important. Total caloric intake influences risk, i.e., imbalance between consumption and expenditure, expecially when (as in industrialized populations) the diet tends to be high in saturated fats and cholesterol. The consequence is not only obesity - a common phenomenon among adults in developed countries, even among children and teenagers in the United States - but frequently also obesity-related hypertriglyceridemic hypercholesterolemia, hypertension, hyperglycemia and hyperuricemia, all implicated as risk factors for atherosclerotic disease.

With this point clearly before us, let us first review the extensive evidence from epidemiologic research on the significance of habitual diet in the etiology of the twentieth century epidemic of coronary disease in the economically advanced countries. Studies of three types have been done on human populations:

1. Analyses of data on nutrition and mortality patterns
   among the nations, as published in reports of the Food
   and Agriculture Organization (FAO) and the World Health
   Organization (WHO);
2. Analyses of autopsy findings from different countries;
3. Field investigations of representative population samples.

While the decisive work has been done since World War II, investigations early in the century had already pointed the way to
the conclusions now firmly established. Thus, a major review in
the pathology literature in the 1930's arrived at the following
generalization, based on an analysis of 28 papers then in the literature, including findings from clinical and pathologic studies
in China, East Africa, Egypt, India, Malaya, Austria, Germany, the
United States, and elsewhere: "In no race for which a high cholesterol intake (in the form of eggs, butter and milk) and fat intake are recorded is atherosclerosis absent.... Where a high protein diet is consumed, which naturally contains small quantities
of cholesterol, but where the neutral fat intake is low, atherosclerosis is not prevalent" (5). Six analyses of FAO-WHO data -
published during the last 25 years - reinforce this conclusion
(6-11). An example of such data from our own studies is presented
in Fig. 1 (10).

Illuminating data are also available from the two other types
of international studies, one utilizing autopsy material, and the
other involving follow-up of representative samples of the living
population - as well as from animal-experimental studies (4). The
International Atherosclerosis Project is the most comprehensive
and systematic study of postmortem findings on aorta and coronary
atherosclerosis in different populations (12). This Project quanti-
tated the degree of atherosclerosis of the aorta and coronary arteries at autopsy in over 31,000 persons age 10 to 69 who died during
1960 to 1965 in 15 cities throughout the world. Marked geographic
differences were recorded in the occurrence of severe atherosclerosis. Significant correlations were found among intake of fat, serum cholesterol level, and severity of coronary atherosclerosis at
autopsy for the populations from the 15 cities.

The International Cooperative Study on the Epidemiology of
Cardiovascular Disease has yielded key data on the role of diet
(13). This prospective international study of 18 population samples in seven countries - Finland, Greece, Italy, Japan, Netherlands, United States, and Yugoslavia - deals with observations on
approximately 12,000 men, originally age 40 to 59, who have been
studied for about a decade. Marked differences in the prevalence
and incidence of coronary heart disease were recorded among the
population samples from seven countries.

Nutrient	Mortality		
	All causes	CHD	CV
Calories, daily total	-.013	.574[c]	.425[a]
Total fat, grams daily	-.089	.472[a]	.265
Total fat, % of calories	-.111	.391	.156
Saturated fat, grams daily	.048	.584[c]	.416
Saturated fat, % of calories	.045	.546[b]	.350
Polyunsaturated fat, grams daily	-.328	-.187	-.335
Polyunsaturated fat, % of calories	-.202	-.340	-.456[a]
Cholesterol, milligrams daily	.098	.626[c]	.534[b]

[a] p = .05; [b] p = .02; [c] p = .01 or less.

Fig. 1. Correlations of nutrients and mortality rates, 22 countries, males 45-54, 1964 (10).

Amount and type of lipid habitually eaten - especially saturated fat, a,d inevitably cholesterol - varied markedly among the
population samples studied (Fig. 2) (13). Thus, in Kyushu, Japan,
total fat constituted 9 per cent of calories, saturated fat 3 per
cent, and polyunsaturated fat 3 per cent. In several of the Euro-
pean communities - e.g., the Greek islands of Corfu and Crete;
Velika Krsna and Dalmatia, Yugoslavia; Montegiorgio and Crevalcore,
Italy - saturated fat intake was also low (7 to 10 per cent of calories); polyunsaturated fat intake was never high (3 to 7 per cent).
(For some of these southern Europe populations consuming considerable olive oil, total fat made up as much as 40 per cent of calories, but saturated fat intake was still low, as was polyunsaturated fat intake, since olive oil is composed largely of mono-unsaturated oleic acid). In contrast, analyses of the diets ingested by the men under study in Finland, the Netherlands, and the
United States revealed high saturated fat intakes, in the range
of 17 to 22 per cent of calories (total fat 35 to 40 percent, polyunsaturated fat 3 to 5 per cent). Men from East Finland exhibited the highest levels of saturated fat ingestion - 22 per cent of
total calories.

As shown in the Fig. 3, saturated fat intake and 5 year incidence rates of coronary heart disease for these population samples showed a high order positive correlation that was statistically significant (13).

Saturated fat intake and serum cholesterol level of the populations were highly and significantly correlated (Fig. 4). In
turn, cholesterol and incidence rates were highly and significantly correlated (Fig. 5) (13).

Most of the other components of the analyzed diets - total
calories, total fat, mono-unsaturated fat, polyunsaturated fat,
total protein - were not significantly related to serum cholesterol
levels or coronary heart disease incidence rates of the cohorts.
Dietary cholesterol was not systematically evaluated. Sucrose intake - significantly correlated with saturated fat intake - was
significantly correlated with coronary heart disease incidence
($r = 0.78$). However, when this analysis was extended beyond simple correlation, with consideration simultaneously to both saturated fat and sucrose, the association between saturated fat intake
and CHD incidence remained highly significant statistically, that
between sucrose and CHD incidence became insignificant (14).

Recently, one investigator in particular has emphasized the
positive correlation between sucrose intake and incidence rates
for coronary heart disease (15). He has invoked for sucrose a
major, primary, and specific role in atherogenesis. This issue
has been reviewed at length elsewhere, and its detailed examination
is beyond the scope of this presentation (14,16,17). Suffice it

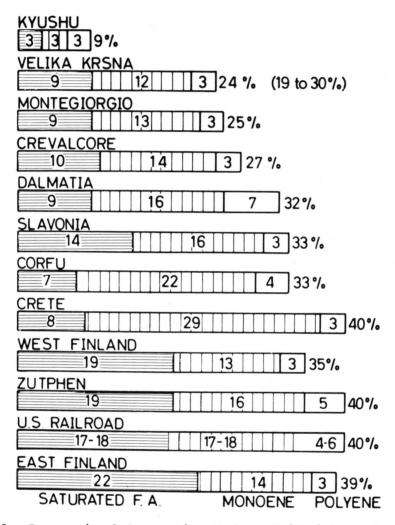

Fig. 2.   International Cooperative Study on Epidemiology of Cardio-vascular Disease; average percentage of dietary calories provided by saturated, mono-ene, and polysaturated fatty acids (13).

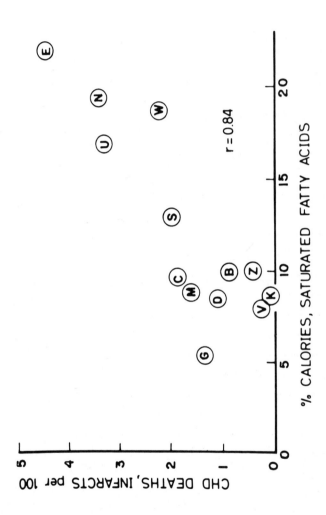

Fig. 3. International Cooperative Study on Epidemiology of Cardiovascular Disease; men originally age 40-59 in seven countries; relationship between percentage of total calories provided by
saturated fatty acids in the diet of the cohorts and age-standardized 5-year incidence rate for
fatal coronary heart disease plus non-fatal myocardial infarction. The cohorts are:
E= East Finland; U=U.S. railroad; W= West Finland; N= Zutphen, the Netherlands;
C= Crevalcore, Italy; M= Montegiorgio, Italy; S= Slavonia, Yugoslavia; B= Belgrade, Yugoslavia;
Z= Zrenjanin, Yugoslavia; D= Dalmatia, Yugoslavia; V= Velika Krsna, Yugoslavia; G= Corfu, Greece;
K= Crete, Greece (13).

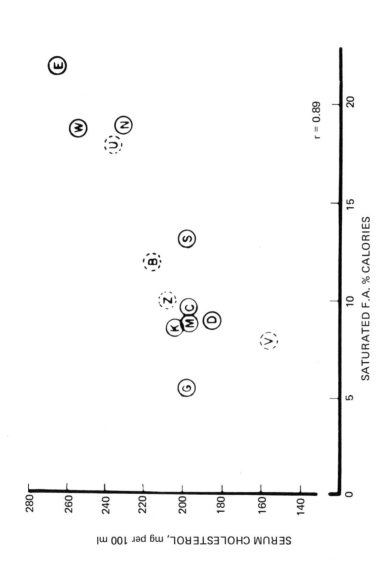

Fig. 4. International Cooperative Study on Epidemiology of Cardiovascular Disease; relationship between average percent of total calories from saturated fatty acids in the diet of the cohorts and median serum cholesterol value, as determined at initial examination; men originally age 40–59 in seven countries. For identification of cohorts, see legend for Fig. 3 (13).

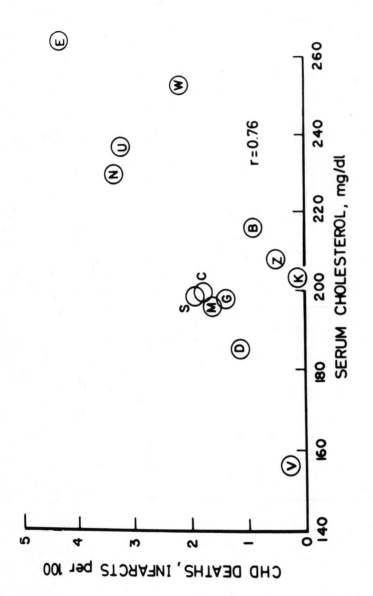

Fig. 5. International Cooperative Study on Epidemiology of Cardiovascular Disease; relationship between median cholesterol concentration for the cohorts at initial examination and age-standardized 5-year incidence rate for fatal coronary heart disease plus non-fatal myocardial infarction; men originally age 40-59 in seven countries. For identification of cohorts, see legend for Fig. 3 (13).

to note here that several major sets of evidence - animal-experimental, clinical and epidemiologic - render untenable the hypothesis that sucrose is a prime and decisive factor influencing atherogenesis.

Extensive data are also available from hundreds of studies, using a diversity of research methodologies indicating that the correlations between lipid intake (saturated fat, cholesterol) and coronary heart disease rates are indeed highly indicative of independent cause-and-effect relationships. It is valid at the present time to conclude that - at a very high level of probability - an independent cause-and-effect relationship has been demonstrated between dietary lipid (specifically, saturated fat and cholesterol) and widespread, premature coronary heart disease, even though substantial direct proof from definitive, large-scale, long-term mass field trials is still to be obtained (see below). This conclusion is almost certainly valid since: data on the epidemiologic associations are available from many sources; the associations persist when confounding variables are taken into account; are strongly consistent; are in harmony with findings from other research methods (i.e., animal esperimentation and clinico-pathologic investigation); are coherent in terms of reasonable pathogenetic mechanisms relating apparent causes and the disease (see below); and all alternative hypotheses purporting to account for the nutritional aspects of the etiology of premature atherosclerotic disease (e.g., the polyunsaturated fat deficiency and the high sucrose hypotheses) are invalidated by the totality of the data. This conclusion of course, does not mean that dietary lipid composition is the sole cause of the current epidemic of premature, severe atherosclerotic disease. It does mean that habitual high intake of saturated fat and cholesterol is a key, primary, indispensible etiologic factor in the epidemic.

One of the most important research advances since World War II is the delineation of the chief mechanism of the etiologic effect of dietary lipid on atherogenesis. This has been the demonstration - as illustrated in the last three figures - that populations differing in habitual intake of saturated fat and cholesterol also differ markedly in serum cholesterol levels, i.e., interpopulation levels of these two sets of variables are highly correlated. So also are dietary saturated fat-cholesterol intake and coronary heart rates, and serum cholesterol level and coronary heart disease rates.

As is evident from these figures, the variables used to characterize the populations with respect to nutrients and cholesterolemia are means or medians. For these interpopulation comparisons, the range of values within each population - i.e., the interindividual variation - is ignored.

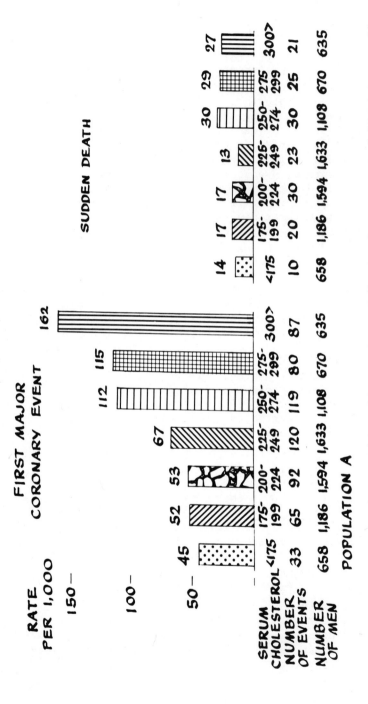

Fig. 6. National Cooperative Pooling Project; serum cholesterol at entry and 10-year age-adjusted rates per 1,000 men for: first major coronary event and sudden death (upper graph), any coronary death and death from all causes (lower graph); first major coronary event includes non-fatal myocardial infarction, fatal myocardial infarction and sudden death due to CHD; U.S. white males age 30-59 at entry; all rates age-adjusted by 10-year age groups to the U.S. white male population, 1960 (4).

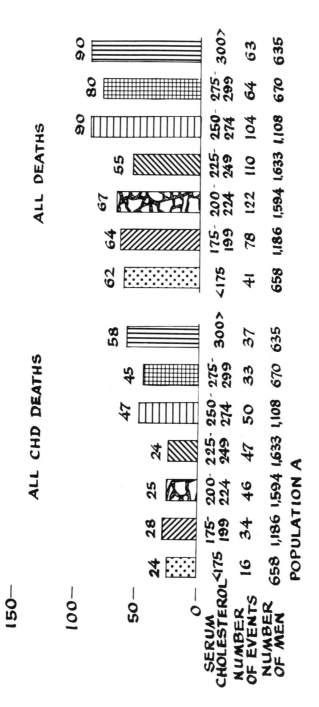

Fig. 6. (lower graph) See Legend of Fig. 6. (upper graph).

For any single population, interindividual variation in nu-
trient ingestion (e.g., saturated fat) is generally small. Nevertheless, a large interindividual variation exists in serum cholesterol levels - its mechanisms in intermediary metabolism still
largely unknown (3). This wide interindividual variation in serum
cholesterol levels within a population permits a further evaluation
- in addition to the earlier cited interpopulation evaluation - of
the relationship between serum cholesterol and risk of atherosclerotic disease. Extensive data on this matter are available, particularly in relation to premature coronary heart disease in the
United States. They are summarized in Fig. 6, from the national
cooperative Pooling Project, involving pooled data from several
long-term prospective studies of United States males (4). In the
analysis of these data use was made of only the first serum cholesterol determination, done at the time of initial examination.
Thus, this analysis suffered from all the difficulties of a single
measurement, particularly intra-individual fluctuation and laboratory analytical error. Nevertheless, highly significant relationships are clearly evident between serum cholesterol level and risk
of major coronary events.

The available data further indicate that for United States
white males age 40-44, 45-49, 50-54, 55-59, and 60-64, relative
risk remains substantial even for the oldest age group. Absolute
excess risk remains the same or even increases with age. Absolute
excess risk is the probability of experiencing a heart attack in
any given year for a man in a higher quintile compared to one in
the lowest quintile (risk of the former minus risk of the latter).
From the point of view of the individual patient, and his physician, absolute risk and absolute excess risk are the decisive matters. Clearly, these data indicate the potential value of identi-
fying and **correcting** hypercholesterolemia by safe means, beginning as early in life as possible, for purposes of primary prevention.

Recent data from the Coronary Drug Project indicate that serum cholesterol level remains predictive of risk of dying for men
who have recovered from one or more myocardial infarctions in middle age (18,19). This new finding confirms that there is also a
substantial rationale for treatment of hypercholesterolemia in patients with frank clinical coronary heart disease, for purposes
of secondary prevention.

Finally, data from the Framingham study indicate that for
male decedents at autopsy, serum cholesterol measurements made
5 and 9 years prior to death were significantly correlated with
severity of coronary atherosclerosis, as measured by both percent
intimal involvement and per cent luminal insufficiency (20).

Clearly, the evidence on the association between serum cholesterol level and atherosclerosis is extensive and powerful.

The amassed data further demonstrate incontrovertibly that
there is a steady increment in premature atherosclerotic disease
as level of serum cholesterol rises. As cholesterol concentration increases, risk increases. The relationship is continuous.
This is true at all ages, at least from young adulthood through
middle age. There is no evidence of a critical level which di-
vides "normal" subgroups (i.e., subgroups "immune" to premature
coronary disease) from coronary heart disease-prone "abnormal"
subgroups. Nor is there any justification for using the Gaussian
distribution to define "normal" levels. It is unfortunate that
this distribution was named the "normal curve" by statisticians.
They had no intent to imply anything about biologic or medical
normalcy. Yet right up to the present this distribution – and
particularly the level two standard deviations above the mean in
our population – is being used to define upper limit of biological
normal for specific age-sex groups. This is an unjustifiable definition of normal based on what exists – what is prevalent – in
a population, without regard to the continuous relationship between serum cholesterol and risk, and without regard to the lessons
from comparative studies of other human populations and other species.

For the physician responsible for patients, the basic facts
about the continuous relationship between serum cholesterol level
and risk are of the utmost practical importance with regard to
prescribing measures for prevention. The greater the probability,
the greater the need for prophylaxis – but there is no single
"screening level" separating those in need of prophylaxis from
those who are not.

This basic set of conclusions does not negate – but rather
places in proper context – the clinical use of practical cutting
points, e.g., serum cholesterol of less than 200 mg per dl as normal, 200 to 249 as borderline, 250 or greater as abnormal for
adults age 30 and over. This 250 mg per dl level for defining
hypercholesterolemia is approximately the 2 to 1 cutting point,
i.e., persons positive for this risk factor are approximately
twice as susceptible to premature coronary heart disease as those
with lower levels (everything else being equal). The impact of
these factors is no small 10 per cent, but rather 100 per cent –
a doubling of risk. But as useful as this practical approach of
cutting points is, it remains a distortion of reality. After all,
a person with a serum cholesterol of 240 is at greater risk than
one at 210, and this person in turn is at greater risk than one
at 160.

Moreover, a serum cholesterol level of 240 has an entirely
different risk impact for a pack-a-day cigarette smoker with a
diastolic blood pressure of 96, than for a nonsmoker with a pressure of 74 mm Hg (4). At present, techniques for multivariate
risk function analysis are becoming available to physicians, to

permit them to evaluate risk factors simultaneously, as continuous quantitative variables (21). These are a useful improvement over previous approaches - already valuable - for assessing the significance of serum cholesterol level and quantitating susceptibility to premature atherosclerotic disease.

As to other serum lipid and lipoprotein measurements and their relationship to risk of atherosclerotic disease, until a year or two ago only three sets of definitive data - i.e., from long-term prospective studies - were available for a scientific assessment (22-24). A fourth has recently been published, with data from Sweden on serum cholesterol and fasting triglycerides as predictors (25). These data show that serum cholesterol and low density lipoprotein (LDL, betalipoprotein, S_f 0-12 and 12-20 lipoprotein) are highly correlated - inevitably, since LDL is the main bearer of serum cholesterol. Correspondingly, serum cholesterol and LDL are about equal as predictors of risk of premature coronary heart disease. Further the first three of these studies indicate that once determination of serum cholesterol has been made, little or nothing is apparently added to predictive power by measurement of very low density lipoprotein (VLDL, prebetalipoprotein, S_f 200-400 lipoprotein) - and therefore of serum triglycerides (VLDL being the main carrier of serum triglycerides). On the other hand, the report from Sweden concludes that fasting serum triglycerides are independently and additively predictive, although - in the judgment of this writer - the published data do not necessarily warrant this inference.

It is very possible that hyperprebetalipoproteinemia has significance for atherogenesis chiefly - perhaps solely - because of the associated hypercholesterolemia. Little evidence is available indicating that - in the absence of hypercholesterolemia - hypertriglyceridemia (whether from endogenously synthesized VLDL molecules or from absorbed chylomicrons) is associated with intensified atherogenesis. Evidence is available - although it is not conclusive - indicating that both LDL and VLDL molecules are atherogenic, the former more so. This is not surprising, in view of recent data confirming that the smaller LDL molecules infiltrate across the arterial intima more readily than the larger VLDL particles, are subject to entrapment in the subintimal tissue (owing in part, at least, to their electrical charge), and bring into this tissue a much greater amount of cholesterol (especially cholesterol ester) than VLDL per molecule (3). And it is this cholesterol from the plasma, especially cholesterol ester that accumulates in excess - 10-fold, 40-fold above normal levels - as an integral part of atherogenesis, in smooth muscle cells, then (as these disintegrate due to lipid overloading) in extracellular pools, acting as tissue irritants to stimulate scarification (i.e., the sclerotic component of the pathologic process).

On the basis of currently available data, therefore, serum cholesterol is the best single measurement for assessing risk of premature atherosclerotic disease, particularly coronary heart disease. Fasting serum triglycerides or lipoprotein (e.g., as determined qualitatively by paper electrophoresis) are not superior predictors of risk. Earlier claims of this kind, based on preliminary or unsatisfactory data, have not withstood the test of time.

In the management of hypercholesterolemic patients, on the other hand, fasting serum triglyceride determination is a useful adjunct to cholesterol measurement. It is also worthwhile, when the fasting serum is lactescent, to re-examine it after 24 hours in the refrigerator, to determine if a supranatant chylomicron layer is present. In this way, the rare chylomicronemias can readily be ruled out. Of course, the patient must indeed have fasted for 15 hours, after a meal moderate in fat and free of (or low in) alcohol. Otherwise, abnormal chylomicronemia may be erroneously diagnosed. Whether, in addition to these procedures, serum lipoprotein typing (e.g., by electrophoresis) is also worthwhile for clinical management is at present unclear - claims to the contrary notwithstanding.

In the general population, the common phenomenon is "moderate" hypercholesterolemia, either without hypertriglyceridemia, or with slight, moderate, or marked hypertriglyceridemia but without chylomicronemia. (A reasonable cutting point for fasting serum triglyceride abnormality is 150 mg per dl) Once factors known to induce hyperlipidemia (e.g., uncontrolled diabetes, hyperthyroidism, nephrosis, biliary obstruction, pancreatic disease, alcoholism, myeloma, contraceptive steroids) have been ruled out, it may be concluded that the abnormality is fundamentally diet-induced, i.e., acquired, and it can almost always be alleviated by change in diet habits, i.e., to a calorie-controlled diet low in saturated fat and cholesterol, moderate (not low) in total fat and carbohydrate, moderate (not high) in polyunsaturated fat.

To designate the hyperlipidemia common in populations eating a "rich" diet as acquired is not to say that genetic factors are not operating. Since some (a small minority) of persons maintain very low levels of all serum lipids on such diets, there must be an element of host response in all cases of acquired hyperlipidemia, and almost certainly this often reflects inborn (genetic) differences in metabolism. Correspondingly, changing living habits (the environment) on a family basis, to control hereditable risk factors and thereby mute or negate genetic predisposition to premature coronary heart disease is a key aspect of the strategy of focusing on risk factors, to curb the epidemic occurrence of this disease.

Especially for populations from countries with the nutritional prerequisites for premature severe atherosclerosis, elevated blood pressure - in addition to serum cholesterol - is a powerful risk

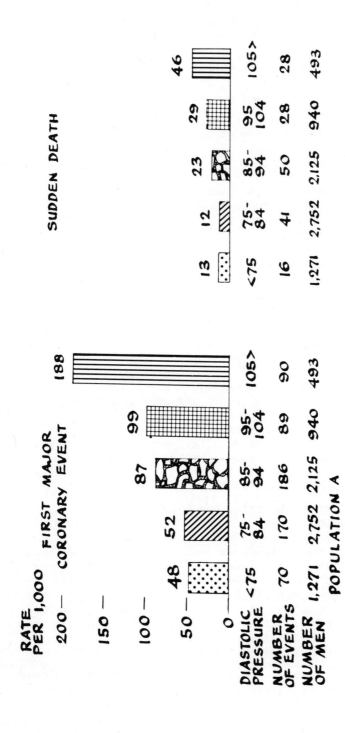

Fig. 7. National Cooperative Pooling Project; diastolic blood pressure level at entry and 10-year age-adjusted rates per 1,000 men for: first major coronary event and sudden death (upper graph), any coronary death, stroke death, death from all causes (lower graph); first major coronary event includes non-fatal myocardial infarction, fatal myocardial infarction, sudden death due to CHD; U.S. white males age 30-59 at entry; all rates age-adjusted by 10-year age groups to the U.S. white male population, 1960 (4).

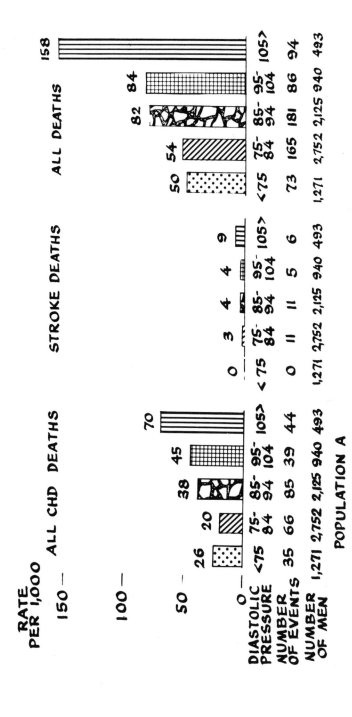

Fig. 7. (lower graph) See Legend of Fig. 7. (upper graph).

factor for atherosclerotic disease, and hypertension has been linked to habitual diet in at least two ways: via the obesity-hyperten-
sion correlation, and via high salt intake. Whatever the limitations of knowledge concerning the etiology of essential hypertension,
and the mechanisms whereby weight reduction of the obese and salt
diuresis lower elevated blood pressure, the unequivocal fact remains that hypertension is a major factor contributing to the epidemic of premature atherosclerotic disease. The autopsy data of
the International Atherosclerosis Project demonstrated a significant relationship between hypertension and the severity of atherosclerosis (12).

Data from the International Cooperative Study on the Epidemiology of Cardiovascular Disease indicate that interpopulation differences in 5 years incidence rates for coronary heart disease are attributable in part to differences in prevalence of hypertension
among the 18 samples of middle-aged men (13).

Data from Americans, from the national cooperative Pooling
Project - on interindividual differences in diastolic blood pressure and their relationship to risk of morbidity and mortality over
the next 10 years - are presented in Fig. 7 (4). Correspondingly
data for systolic pressure show a similar relationship to risk.

The data of the prospective studies demonstrate that at least
for affluent populations hypertension is related to risk of premature
coronary disease independent of and additive to the impact of such
other major risk factors as hypercholesterolemia and cigarette smoking. In fact, the impact of all three of these major risk factors
is additive - as shown in Fig. 8, from the national cooperative
Pooling Project (4). It deals with various combinations of hypercholesterolemia, hypertension, and cigarette smoking. Several features of these data are noteworthy. First, the analysis is a simple and crude one, in that only a single measurement at entry examination is utilized to characterize each man, and his status with
respect to the specific risk factors was based on dichomotization
of the data, utilizing the specified cutting points. Obviously,
a serum cholesterol level of 240 mg per dl is by no means an optimal level, in terms of risk, and similarly with respect to diastolic blood pressure of 88 mm Hg. Nevertheless, for purposes of this
analysis, such values were designated "not high".

At all ages, presence of only one risk factor - as compared
to none - was associated with a substantial increase in probability
of a major event over the next years. When combinations of risk
factors - any two or all three - were present, susceptibility to
overt coronary heart disease was substantially higher, attaining
levels many times greater than for the group with none of the
three risk factors present. These high levels of excess risk -
both relative and absolute - are present for men with these combinations of factors at all ages at least through the 60-64 range.

Obviously, it is highly appropriate to designate persons with such combinations of these traits as very high risk individuals, very prone to developing premature atherosclerotic disease.

As already indicated, modern mathematical methods for multi-factorial analysis of risk further enhance our ability to quantitate coronary-proneness to development of coronary heart disease (3,21).

For years, it has been recognized that persons with clinically diagnosed diabetes mellitus are at serious risk of developing atherosclerotic disease. However, the mechanism of this association remains obscure. Recently epidemiologic research has been exploring this problem, with a focus on the key question: Is hyperglycemia (glucose-intolerance) per se a risk factor for atherosclerotic disease, or - more precisely, is it a risk factor independent of and additive to the major factors ("rich" diet, hypercholesterolemic hyperlipidemia, hypertension, cigarette smoking). (As already noted, risk of hyperglycemia is itself diet-related, insofar as chronic caloric imbalance with resultant obesity is associated with greater proneness to glucose intolerance).

Abundant data from univeriate analyses confirm that hyperglycemia and atherosclerotic disease are associated. The data from the Chicago Heart Association's large scale Detection Project in Industry (Fig. 9) further confirm this simple relationship (26-29). As one goes up the scale of plasma glucose level 1-hour after a 50 gm oral load, the rate of major ECG abnormalities becomes higher, this being especially conspicuous for the group with levels of 205 and greater - and for three of the four major age-sex groups, the relationship is significant statistically. However, matters are by no means so clearcut and definitive when the risk factors which correlate with plasma glucose, are considered simultaneously in multivariate analyses. This is particularly true when the confounding effects of medication for hypertension and/or hyperglycemia are controlled in the analysis.

Fig. 10 illustrates the results of a multifactor cross-classification analysis from the same study, for white men age 45-64, with five risk factors dichotomized (including plasma glucose 1-hour post-50-gm-oral-load). With exclusion from the analysis of hypertensives on treatment and diabetics on treatment, glucose and rate of major ECG abnormalities were significantly related in two cases (noted by asterisks), but not in two others, and in only one of four comparisons for white women age 45-64 (Fig. 11). Similar inconsistent results were obtained with the more elegant multiple logistic regression technique (Fig. 12) where in only two of four analyses (after exclusion of hypertensives on treatment) were the values greater than 2.00 obtained indicating a significant relationship between post-load plasma glucose and major ECG abnormalities. Another recent Chicago cross-sectional study of 10,000 people has

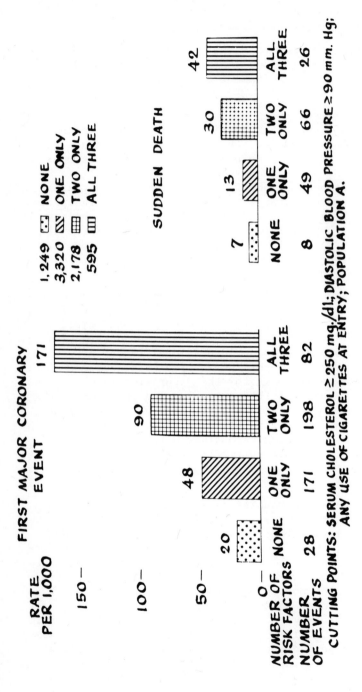

Fig. 8. National Cooperative Pooling Project; hypercholesterolemia, hypertension, cigarette smoking and 10-year age-adjusted rates per 1,000 men for: first major coronary event, sudden death (upper graph), any coronary death, death from all causes (lower graph); first major coronary event includes non-fatal myocardial infarction, fatal myocardial infarction and sudden death due to CHD; U.S. white males age 30–59 at entry; all rates age-adjusted by 10-year age groups to the U.S. white male population, 1960 (4).

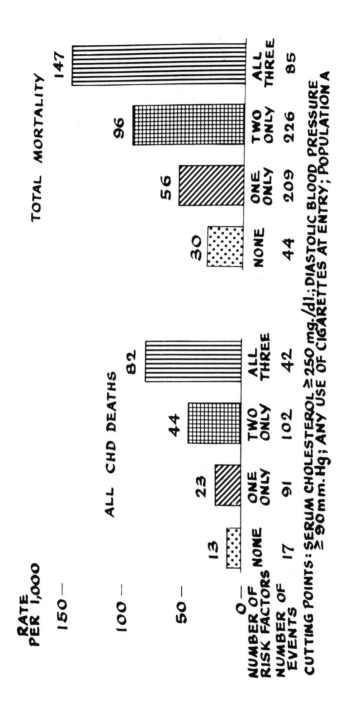

Fig. 8. (lower graph) See Legend of Fig. 8. (upper graph).

ONE-HOUR POST-LOAD PLASMA GLUCOSE	PERSONS AGE 25-44				PERSONS AGE 45-64			
	WHITE MALE		WHITE FEMALE		WHITE MALE		WHITE FEMALE	
	NO.	RATE/1,000	NO.	RATE/1,000	NO.	RATE/1,000	NO.	RATE/1,000
<85	758	19	423	52	178	21	245	93
85-124	4,493	22	2,026	50	1,737	60	1,894	92
125-164	2,685	20	1,155	69	2,264	64	1,936	97
165-204	965	22	410	72	1,278	63	946	130
≥205	321	36	102	216	784	124	525	146
ALL	9,222	21	4,116	60**	6,241	70**	5,546	106△

RATE AGE-ADJUSTED BY 5-YEAR AGE GROUPS TO CORRESPONDING SEX GROUP OF U.S. WHITE POPULATION, 1960.
** SLOPE SIGNIFICANTLY DIFFERENT FROM O AT .02 LEVEL.
△ SLOPE SIGNIFICANTLY DIFFERENT AT .05 LEVEL.   1967-1972

Fig. 9. Chicago Heart Association Detection Project in Industry; one-hour post-load plasma glucose and rate of ECG myocardial infarction, ischemia, or current of injury patterns, whites by age-sex, exclusive of those on antihypertensive medication (29).

Risk Factors	No Exclusions		Excludes Hyp. on Rx and Diab. on Rx	
	N	R/1000	N	R/1000
None of 5	1,158	35	1,120	34
Glucose Only	113	53	88	56
1 Only of 4	2,204	68	2,075	59
1 Only of 4 + Glucose	319	115**	239	115*
2 Only of 4	1,752	86	1,574	70
2 Only of 4 + Glucose	413	148***	314	140***
3 or 4 (of 4)	749	115	672	93
3 or 4 (of 4) + G	201	183*	139	140

Glucose $\geq$ 205, Chol. $\geq$ 250, DBP $\geq$ 90,
Any Cigarettes, Rel. Wt. $\geq$ 1.25.

Fig. 10. Chicago Heart Association Detection Project in Industry; plasma glucose, other risk factors and myocardial infarction, ischemia, digitalis effect, current of injury, white males age 45–64 (29).

Risk Factors	No Exclusions		Excludes Hyp. on Rx and Diab. on Rx	
	N	R/1000	N	R/1000
None of 5	1,286	85	1,229	76
Glucose Only	99	163	83	121
1 Only of 4	2,198	102	2,057	93
1 Only of 4 + Glucose	255	164**	195	125
2 Only of 4	1,478	141	1,288	130
2 Only of 4 + Glucose	224	192	161	143
3 or 4 (of 4)	528	145	424	127
3 or 4 (of 4) + G	119	208	81	223*

Glucose $\geq$ 205, Chol. $\geq$ 250, DBP $\geq$ 90,
Any Cigarettes, Rel. Wt. $\geq$ 1.25.

Fig. 11. Chicago Heart Association Detection Project in Industry; plasma glucose, other risk factors and myocardial infarction, ischemia, digitalis effect, current of injury; white females, age 45-64 (29).

SEX – AGE	INCLUSIVE OF PERSONS ON ANTIHYPERTENSIVE ℞			EXCLUSIVE OF PERSONS ON ANTIHYPERTENSIVE ℞		
	NO. OF PERSONS	NO. OF EVENTS	t VALUE FOR GLUCOSE	NO. OF PERSONS	NO. OF EVENTS	t VALUE FOR GLUCOSE
MALE 25-44	9,315	205	.23	9,169	190	-.30
MALE 45-64	6,748	513	3.01	6,221	403	2.99
FEMALE 25-44	4,147	259	2.96	4,075	247	3.66
FEMALE 45-64	6,106	716	3.12	5,518	568	1.48

Fig. 12. Chicago Heart Association Detection Project in Industry; one-hour post-load plasma glucose and myocardial infarction, ischemia, current of injury on ECG; 7 variable multiple logistic regression analysis, by age-sex, whites, including and excluding persons on antihypertensive treatment. The seven variables are: age, cigarettes per day, systolic blood pressure, diastolic blood pressure, serum cholesterol, relative weight, 1-hour post-load plasma glucose (29).

yielded similar inconclusive data, and review of the few sets of data available from other groups also indicate uncertainties (30). In sum, basic questions remain to be clarified: Is hyperglycemia an independent and additive risk factor for atherosclerotic disease? What are the mechanisms - over and above chronic caloric imbalance - of the associations between hyperglycemia and hyperlipidemia, between hyperglycemia and hypertension? Is a good deal of the excess atherosclerosis risk of mild maturity-onset nonketotic non-insulin-dependent diabetes in our population a result of the concomitant hypertension and/or hyperlipidemia, and not independently related to hyperglycemia per se?

The posing of these questions is not an esoteric exercise in epidemiologic dialectics. Very practical issues are involved. Diabetics of this type number in the millions if widely-accepted present-day criteria for glucose intolerance are valid - e.g., an estimated 10,000,000 in the United States - and their prime problem is risk of atherosclerotic "complications". It has been reaffirmed by the results of the University Group Diabetes Program study that treatment of hyperglycemia with drugs - oral or parenteral (insulin) - is ineffective in averting morbidity or mortality from cardiovascular complications in such diabetics (31,32). Their atherosclerosis is no different in kind, but only in degree, from that of nondiabetics. Therefore a total reconsideration and redefinition is needed of control for such diabetics. Even if for practical purposes we assume - or, rather, especially if we assume - that hyperglycemia is an independent and additive coronary heart disease risk factor for the diabetic, his risk of premature atherosclerotic disease is also potently related to his blood pressure, serum cholesterol, cigarette smoking - i.e., to the major coronary risk factors. Therefore control cannot remain focussed narrowly on blood and urine glucose, but must become comprehensive. It must include effective control of obesity, to correct hyperglycemia and hypertension, as well as attention to fat composition of the diet, to correct hyperlipidemia. And cigarette smoking must also be corrected. Hope for the prevention of atherosclerotic disease in diabetics lies only in such a comprehensive approach to control.

In conclusion, it is relevant to return to the opening theme: our concern for diet-dependent risk factors as they relate to the epidemic of atherosclerotic disease in the developed countries.

Study of the history of epidemic diseases - e.g., typhus, plague, cholera, tuberculosis, pellagra - yields a basic generalization: epidemic disease occurs in populations when socioeconomic and sociocultural developments engender a confluence of multiple causes essential for the massive onslaught of sickness (3). The decisive role of socioeconomic and sociocultural factors in the genesis of epidemics was identified over a century ago by one of the great founders of modern scientific medicine, Rudolf Virchow:

> "Don't crowd diseases point everywhere to deficiencies
> of society? One may adduce atmospheric or cosmic con-
> ditions or similar factors. But never do they alone
> make epidemics. They produce them only there where
> due to bad social conditions people have lived for
> some time in abnormal situations".

> "Epidemics of a character unknown so far appear, and
> often disappear without traces when a new culture
> period has started. Thus did leprosy and the English
> sweat. The history of artificial epidemics is there-
> fore the history of disturbances of human culture.
> Their changes announce to us in gigantic signs the
> turning points of culture into new directions."

> "Epidemics resemble great warning signs on which the
> true statesman is able to read that the evolution of
> his nation has been disturbed to a point which even a
> careless policy is no longer allowed to overlook..."
> (33).

Coronary heart disease has in the course of the twentieth
century replaced tuberculosis as the great epidemic disease of
the era in the industrialized countries. Coronary heart disease
is the epidemic disease of mature, advanced industrial society,
as tuberculosis was the epidemic disease of this society in its
childhood and adolescence.

One key circumstance is that the mass of the population in
affluent countries has for the first time in history been able
to enjoy a "rich" diet high in animal products (meats, dairy foods),
and has not been restricted by harsh economic conditions to cheap
starchy foods (bread, potatoes, pasta, oatmeal, cornmeal, etc.).
This modern diet - excessive in calories in relation to energy expenditure, high in total fat, saturated fat, cholesterol, sugar,
and salt - leads to high prevalence rates of hyperlipidemia (hypercholesterolemia, hypertriglyceridemia, hyperlipoproteinemia) in
the adult population. And sustained hypercholesterolemic hyperlipidemia markedly increases risk of premature severe atherosclerotic
disease and its clinical sequelae.

Important as this etiologic chain of events is, it is not the
exclusive one - let us reemphasize - involving diet in the pathogenesis and causation of the coronary heart disease epidemic. The
modern "rich" diet also contributes significantly to current high
prevalence rates of obesity, and consequently of hypertension,
hyperglycemia, and hyperuricemia - and all of these have also been
implicated as coronary risk factors. Thus diet is related to the
coronary heart disease epidemic through at least four etiopatho-
genic mechanisms, and not just one.

A second circumstance, the other side (so to speak) of the coin of "rich" diet, is the emergence of a sedentary mode of living and poor cardiopulmonary fitness as mass phenomena in the twentieth century - as a result of greater and greater use of nonhuman energy in large-scale production, the motor car, television, and so forth. In most industrialized countries, man no longer has to "earn his bread by the sweat of his brow" - and he doesn't subsist chiefly on bread nowadays! Aside from any other negative effects, this change certainly contributes to chronic caloric imbalance and frequent obesity - e.g., prevalence rates of 20 per cent among teenagers and 50 per cent among middle-aged adults in the United States - with all the consequences. Although the evidence is not entirely airtight and consistent, there is good reason to believe that lack of exercise - habitual inactivity at work and leisure and consequent poor cardiopulmonary fitness - is another important aspect of the modern mode of life, interdigitating with "rich" diet, increasing susceptibility to premature coronary heart disease.

A third aspect of the twentieth century way of life contributing powerfully to the coronary heart disease epidemic has been the mass consumption of cigarettes since World War I. And there is no longer any doubt that cigarette smoking is a major factor adding substantially to risk of coronary heart disease, at least among the populations of the advanced countries, with the nutritional-metabolic prerequisites for atherogenesis.

Finally, available data indicate that the stresses, tensions, and conflicts of modern life in highly urbanized society, the pace, turmoil, mobility, change - and their effects on personality and behavior - act as insult added to injury for sizeable segments of the populations of the advanced countries.

These psychocultural factors, too - along with the "rich" diet, cigarette smoking, sedentary living - seem to be playing an important role in the causation of the coronary heart disease epidemic in the developed countries.

The basic thesis summarized above is that socioeconomic and sociocultural evolution in the advanced countries in thetwentieth century has led to a way of life for tens and hundreds of millions that is conducive to high prevalence rates of major coronary risk factors, including diet-related risk factors, and consequently to high incidence rates of premature coronary disease. That is, high prevalence rates of coronary risk factors - repeatedly recorded at present in populations of the developed countries - are resultants of the contemporary mode of life. They are not bolts from the blue mysteriously striking individuals. Nor are they, in most cases, chiefly genetic in origin. True in a small per cent of the population severe hereditary metabolic dyscrasias are present, leading - for example - to severe hyperlipidemia amenable only in

a limited degree to dietary control. However, this is the exception rather than the rule. For most persons, hyperlipidemia (to
continue the example) is in essence an acquired abnormality – a
resultant primarily of a lifetime diet high in calories, saturated fats, and cholesterol.

Actually, there is always a host factor, the phenomenon is
never purely environmental in origin. This is evident from the
fact that a small per cent of persons eating "rich" diets maintain optimal low levels of all serum lipids throughout adulthood.
The range of serum cholesterol and triglycerides in a given population – e.g., a standard deviation of about 40 to 50 mg per dl
about a mean of 230 to 240 mg for serum cholesterol for United
States middle-aged men – almost certainly is due in large measure
to inborn difference in metabolism (nature unknown).

However, this conclusion in no way contradicts the inference
that in terms of mass phenomena – the high prevalence rates of
coronary risk factors in the adult populations of the developed
countries – the fundamental cause is the mode of life.

This conclusion – with its obvious direct corollary that the
epidemic can be controlled – has important practical consequences:
Changes in diet and mode of life are not only essential to reduce
risk of tens of millions of coronary-prone persons in the adult
population now. They are also vital prerequisites for rearing
upcoming generations with new and better habits, instituted in
infancy, childhood, and adolescence – to assure the disappearance
of now widely prevalent overeating, sedentary living, cigarette
smoking, and resultant commonplace hyperlipidemia, obesity, hypertension, hyperglucemia, hyperuricemia, impaired cardiopulmonary
fitness, etc.

Obviously, whether infants grow up habituated to high-satur-
ated-fat, high-cholesterol, high-calorie diets, to cigarette smoking, to sedentary ways – i.e., whether they acquire life styles
that contribute to susceptibility to premature atherosclerotic
disease is determined largely by familial and social circumstances.
Fundamentally, then, these environmentally conditioned risk factors
are all avoidable. They are amenable first and foremost to primary prevention, i.e., prevention "at the source", through initial
formation of good habits from childhood on, the easiest and most
successful way. Or – if necessary, as is the case en masse in affluent populations today – they are amenable to secondary prevention, i.e., elimination of bad habits and their replacement by
good ones (more difficult, but nonetheless feasible and useful).

As to the risk factors involving endogenous biochemical-phy-
siologic regulatory mechanisms, they too are amenable to exogenous
influences, and can usually be prevented, controlled, corrected,
or ameliorated by changes in mode of life, plus – where necessary

and appropriate - long-term pharmacologic treatment. Thus prevention or control of hypercholesterolemia-hyperlipidemia may be effected for most persons by acceptable modification of the diet.
Weight reduction - especially on a diet low in saturated fat and cholesterol, moderate in sugars, total carbohydrate, unsaturated fat, salt - frequently lowers elevated serum lipids, as well as blood pressure and plasma glucose levels in obese patients. In addition, well-tested pharmacologic measures are available for the control of hypertension not responsive to dietary management alone. Cigarette smoking is also amenable to prevention or correction on a large scale, as shown by recent declines in the proportion of cigarette smokers in the adult American population in general, and among physicians in particular.

Encouraging results are available from several research studies evaluating effects of modifying major risk factors - "rich" diet, hyperlipidemia, hypertension, and cigarette smoking (2-4).
Only such changes - brought about by a steadily mounting, well planned widespread social effort involving the whole population - offer any hope of ending the upward spiral of the coronary heart disease epidemic and effecting a downturn.

ACKNOWLEDGEMENTS

It is a pleasure to acknowledge the cooperation of the author's senior colleagues in the long-term investigations presented here: especially Howard Adler, Ph.D., David M. Berkson, M.D., Alan Dyer, Ph.D., Morton B. Epstein, Ph.D., Yolanda Hall, M.S., Howard A. Lindberg, M.D., Louise Mojonnier, Ph.D., James A. Schoenberger, M.D., Richard B. Shekelle, Ph.D. and Rose Stamer, M.A. It is also a pleasure to express appreciation to the many Chicago organizations giving invaluable cooperation in the cited research efforts, particularly the Chicago Board of Health (Eric Oldberg, M.D., President); Chicago Health Research Foundation (Eric Oldberg, M.D., Chairman); Chicago Heart Association and its Detection Project in Industry (Susan Shekelle, Coordinator); Peoples Gas Light and Coke Company and its Chairman, Remick McDowell.

The author is also most grateful to the principal investigators of the prospective studies of Albany civil servants, Chicago Western Electric Company employees, Framingham community residents, Los Angeles civil servants, and Minneapolis-St. Paul business and professional men, and to the coordinators of the national cooperative Pooling Project. It is a pleasure to acknowledge the cooperation and aid of our colleagues in this endeavor, Drs. Henry Blackburn, John M. Chapman, Thomas R. Dawber, Joseph T. Doyle, Frederick H. Epstein, William B. Kannel, Ancel Keys, Felix J. Moore, Oglesby Paul and Henry Taylor.

Appreciation is also expressed to Professor Ancel Keys and his colleagues of the Seven Countries study, and to the American Heart Association for permission to cite from reports published in Circulation.

The research by our group reported here has been supported by the American Heart Association; Chicago Heart Association; Illinois Regional Medical Program; and the National Heart and Lung Institute, National Institutes of Health, United States Public Health Service.

REFERENCES

1. Katz, L.N., Stamler, J. and Pick, R.P.
   Nutrition and Atherosclerosis, Lea and Febiger,
   Philadelphia, Pa., 1958.
2. Stamler, J.
   Lectures on Preventive Cardiology, Grune and Stratton,
   New York, N.Y., 1967.
3. Stamler, J., Berkson, D.M. and Lindberg, H.A.
   Risk Factors: Their Role in the Etiology and Pathogenesis
   of the Atherosclerotic Diseases.
   Wissler, R.W. and Geer, J.C., eds., Pathogenesis of
   Atherosclerosis, Williams and Wilkins, Baltimore, Md.,
   p. 41, 1972.
4. Inter-Society Commission for Heart Disease Resources.
   Atherosclerosis Study Group and Epidemiology Study Group.
   Primary Prevention of the Atherosclerotic Diseases.
   Circulation, 42: A55, 1970.
5. Rosenthal, S.R.
   Studies in Atherosclerosis: Chemical, Experimental
   and Morphologic.
   Arch. Path., 18: 473, 660 and 827, 1934.
6. Yerushalmy, J. and Hilleboe, H.E.
   Fat in the Diet and Mortality from Heart Disease - A
   Methodological Note.
   New York State J. Med., 57: 2343, 1957.
7. Jolliffe, N. and Archer, M.
   Statistical Associations between International Coronary
   Heart Disease Death Rates and Certain Environmental Factors.
   J. Chron. Dis., 9: 636, 1959.
8. Connor, W.E.
   Dietary Cholesterol and the Pathogenesis of Atherosclerosis.
   Geriatrics, 16: 407, 1961.
9. Yudkin, J.
   Diet and Coronary Thrombosis-Hypothesis and Fact.
   Lancet, 2: 155, 1957.

10. Stamler, J., Stamler, R. and Shekelle, R.
Regional Differences in Prevalence, Incidence and Mortality
from Atherosclerotic Coronary Heart Disease.
de Haas, J.H., Hemker, H.C. and Snellen, H.A., eds.
Ischaemic Heart Disease, Leiden University Press, Leiden,
The Netherlands, p. 84, 1970.

11. Masironi, F.
Dietary Factors and Coronary Heart Disease.
Bull. WHO, 42: 103, 1970.

12. McGill, H.C., Jr. , ed.
Geographic Pathology of Atherosclerosis,
Williams and Wilkins, Baltimore, Md., 1968.

13. Keys, A., ed.
Coronary Heart Disease in Seven Countries.
Circulation, 41: Suppl. 1, 1970.

14. Keys, A.
Letter to the Editors.
Atherosclerosis, 18: 352, 1973.

15. Yudkin, J. and Morland, J.
Sugar Intake and Myocardial Infarction.
Amer. J. Clin. Nutr., 20: 503, 1967.

16. Stamler, J.
Nutrition, Metabolism and Atherosclerosis - A Review of
Data and Theories, and a Discussion of Controversial
Questions. Ingelfinger, F.J., Relman, A.S. and Finland, M.,
eds. Controversy in Internal Medicine, W.B. Saunders Co.,
Philadelphia, Pa., p. 27, 1966.

17. Walker, A.R.P.
Sugar Intake and Coronary Heart Disease.
Atherosclerosis, 14: 137, 1971.

18. Coronary Drug Project Research Group.
Factors Influencing Long-Term Prognosis after Recovery
from Myocardial Infarction - Three-Year Findings of the
Coronary Drug Project.
J. Chron. Dis.,
In press.

19. Coronary Drug Project Research Group.
The Natural History of Myocardial Infarction in the
Coronary Drug Project: Prognostic Importance of
Serum Lipid Levels,
In press.

20. Feinleib, M., Kannel, W.B., Tedeschi, C.G., Landau, T.K.
and Garrison, R.J.
The Relation of Ante Mortem Characteristics to Cardio-
vascular Findings at Necropsy: The Framingham Study.
Paper presented at the Conference on Cardiovascular
Disease Epidemiology, Council on Epidemiology,
American Heart Association, San Diego, Calif.,Mar. 1-2, 1971.

21. Committee on Reduction of Risk of Heart Attack and Stroke,
    American Heart Association.
    Coronary Risk Handbook - Estimating Risk of Coronary Heart
    Disease in Daily Practice,
    American Heart Association, EM620-PE, New York, N.Y., 1973.
22. Gofman, J.W. et al. and Andrus, E.C. et al.
    Evaluation of Serum Lipoprotein and Cholesterol Measurements
    as Predictors of Clinical Complications of a Cooperative
    Study of Lioproteins and Atherosclerosis.
    Circulation, 14: 691, 1956.
23. Kannel, W.B., Castelli, W.P., Gordon, T. and McNamara, P.M.
    Serum Cholesterol, Lipoproteins, and the Risk of Coronary
    Heart Disease: The Framingham Study.
    Ann. Intern. Med., 74: 1, 1971.
24. Cofman, J.W., Young, W. and Tandy, R.
    Ischemic Heart Disease, Atherosclerosis, and Longevity.
    Circulation, 34: 679, 1966.
25. Carlson, L.A. and Böttiger, L.E.
    Ischaemic Heart-Disease in Relation to Fasting Values of
    Plasma Triglycerides and Cholesterol.
    Lancet, 1: 865, 1972.
26. Stamler, J., Schoenberger, J.A., Lindberg, H.A., Shekelle, R.,
    Stoker, J.M., Epstein, M.B., deBoer, L., Stamler, R.,
    Restivo, R., Gray, D. and Cain, W.
    Detection of Susceptibility to Coronary Disease.
    Bull. N.Y. Acad. Med., 45: 1306, 1969.
27. Schoenberger, J.A., Stamler, J., Shekelle, R.B.
    and Shekelle, S.
    Current Status of Hypertension Control in an Industrial
    Population.
    J.A.M.A., 222: 559, 1972.
28. Stamler, J., Schoenberger, J.A., Shekelle, R.B.
    and Stamler, R.
    Hypertension: The Problem and the Challenge.
    The Hypertension Handbook, Merck, Sharp and Dohme,
    West Point, Pa., p. 3, 1974.
29. Stamler, J., Shekelle, R.B., Schoenberger, J.A.
    and Shekelle, S.
    Glycemia and Its Relationships to Other Risk Factors and
    ECG Abnormalities in 35,000 Employed Chicagoans.
    Paper presented at the Conference on Cardiovascular
    Epidemiology, Council on Epidemiology, American Heart
    Association, New Orleans, La., Mar. 12-13, 1973.
30. Stamler, J., Stamler, R. and Berkson, D.M.
    Is Hyperglycemia and Independent and Additive Risk Factor
    for Coronary Heart Disease? - Findings of the Community
    Screening Program of the Chicago Board of Health.
    In preparation.

31. University Group Diabetes Program.
    The University Group Diabetes Program – A Study of the
    Effects of Hypoglycemic Agents on Vascular Complications
    in Patients with Adult-Onset Diabetes.
    Diabetes, 19: 747, 1970.
32. University Group Diabetes Program.
    Effects of Hypoglycemic Agents on Vascular Complications
    in Patients with Adult-Onset Diabetes: IV. A Preliminary
    Report on Phenformin Results.
    J.A.M.A., 217: 777, 1971.
33. Ackerknecht, E.H.
    Rudolf Virchow – Doctor, Statesman, Anthropologist,
    University of Wisconsin Press, Madison, Wisc., 1953.

DIET AND PLASMA LIPIDS

P.H. SCHREIBMAN

The Rockefeller University

New York, N.Y. 10021

I. DIETARY CHOLESTEROL

The amount of cholesterol in the diet <u>does</u> affect blood cholesterol levels. In a recent study by Mattson and colleagues (1),
a liquid formula diet containing 4 different amounts of cholesterol
was fed to over 60 male prisoners. The results clearly show that
for each 100 mg cholesterol per 1000 calorie increment there is a
linear and predictable rise in serum cholesterol. But, these plasma changes are small and do not tell us how much cholesterol is
actually absorbed.

At The Rockefeller University in New York City, Quintao and
colleagues (2) measured cholesterol absorption by 4 different ra-
dioisotope methods. As the dietary cholesterol increased, the
amount of cholesterol absorbed also increased but not in direct
proportion to the amount fed. Thus, the patient who absorbed 1000
mg on a 2500 mg intake absorbed 250 mg on 500 mg intake.

Fig. 1 illustrates the excretion routes for cholesterol. The
liver synthesizes cholesterol and secretes it into the biliary
tract as cholesterol or bile acids. This amounts to somewhat less
than 1 g/day. Minor losses occur in the urine as steroid hormones
and via the skin as sebum and desquanmated epithelial cells. An
important question addressed in Fig. 2 is: how does the cholesterol
absorbed from the diet affect these synthetic and excretory pathways? There are 4 possibilities. First, as a patient changes from
a cholesterol-free to a cholesterol-containing diet his hepatic
cholesterol synthesis may decrease to compensate for the added
exogenous load. Or the liver may simply re-excrete all of this
dietary load plus the endogenously synthesized cholesterol and bile
acids. Unfortunately, there are 2 remaining possibilities, namely,

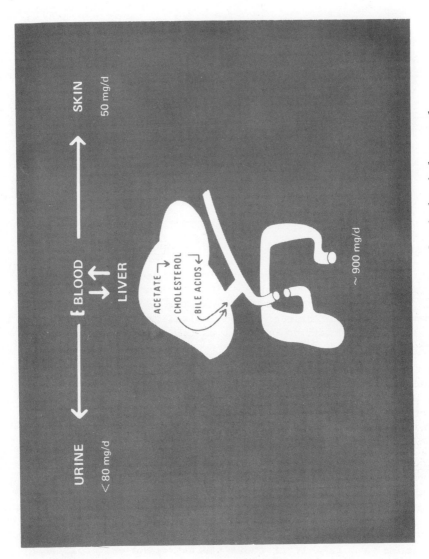

Fig. 1. Excretory routes for body cholesterol.

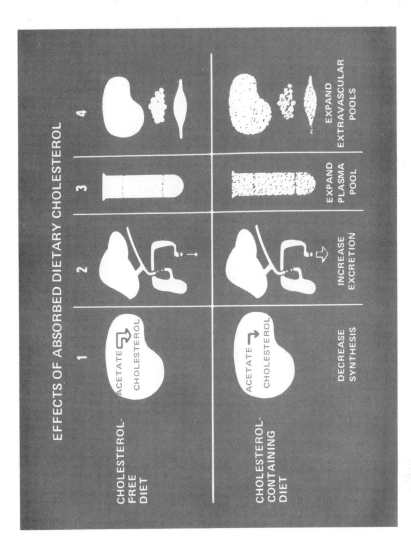

Fig. 2. The two homeostatic mechanisms for maintaining cholesterol balance after absorbing dietary cholesterol are 1) decreasing endogenous synthesis, or 2) increasing fecal excretion. If these are defective then body cholesterol accumulates in either 3) plasma, or 4) extravascular tissues.

that the body will not compensate completely and plasma or extravascular bulk tissues may increase their cholesterol content.
Such an experiment has been performed to determine how different
hyperlipidemic patients actually handle dietary cholesterol.

Eight patients were studied in The Rockefeller University
Hospital (2) for several weeks on cholesterol-free formula diets
and then several weeks on cholesterol-containing diets (Fig. 3).
Measurements of absorption, synthesis and excretion, and plasma
cholesterol concentrations were made in both periods. The response was varied and unpredictable. For example, Patient A absorbed 50 g of cholesterol in some 69 days of cholesterol feeding, re-
excreted 34 g of it in the feces and decreased synthesis by 3 g.
This left 13 g of positive balance of which only 1.1 g of cholesterol accumulated in the plasma. Patient 7, on the other hand absorbed 37 g but almost fully compensated for this by decreasing
endogenous synthesis and re-excreting the absorbed cholesterol.
Two children, with severe familial hypercholesterolemia, Patients
G and H, were not given radio-isotopes so absorption could not be
measured. Nevertheless, they both demonstrated a positive sterol
balance on the dietary cholesterol regime which resulted in a 20
and 22 g cholesterol retention, respectively. Their plasma cholesterol concentrations gave no indication that this had occurred.

II. DIETARY FATTY ACID COMPOSITION

Another dietary factor affecting blood cholesterol concentration is the degree of fatty acid saturation. In carefully controlled studies in many different laboratories, plasma cholesterol
drops consistently when polyunsaturated fat is exchanged isocalorically for saturated fat. A typical experiment is shown in Fig. 4
in which corn oil is substituted for lard. Dietary cholesterol
and plant sterols are constant in both periods. The mechanism
for this effect is still controversial, however. Some investigators find an associated increase in fecal bile acid excretion
(3, 4) whereas other equally expert workers (5, 6) find no significant excretion changes as illustrated in Fig. 4. These workers
hypothesize a shift of cholesterol from plasma to other unknown
tissues. This question is of obvious importance and should be
answered before dietary recommendations are given on an international scale.

III. PLASMA TRIGLYCERIDES

I will now turn to a brief discussion of plasma triglycerides
as a risk factor for atherosclerosis. Recently, Carlson and Böttiger (7) reported on a study of over 3000 men in Stockholm followed for 8 years (Fig. 5). The vertical axis shows the rate of
new heart disease during those years and the horizontal axis groups

DIETARY CHOLESTEROL
AND REGULATION OF BODY CHOLESTEROL (g)

From Quintao, Grundy, and Ahrens, 1971

PATIENT	A	B	C	D	E	F	G	H
TOTAL ABSORPTION	50	44	42	17	15	37	-	-
RE-EXCRETED	34	19	11	4	5	12	-	-
DECREASED SYNTHESIS	3	34	27	8	9	24	-	-
ACCUMULATION	13	−9	4	5	1	1	20	22
RISE IN PLASMA CHOLESTEROL	1.14	1.16	0.82	0.93	−0.96	0.97	−0.27	0.50
PLASMA	1.1	1.2	0.8	0.9	−1.0	1.0	−0.3	0.5
EXTRAVASCULAR	11.9	−7.8	3.2	4.1	2.0	0.0	20.3	19.5

Fig. 3. Modification of Table V, reference 2. The altered sterol balance effects are shown for 8 patients after changing from cholesterol-free to cholesterol-containing formula diets.

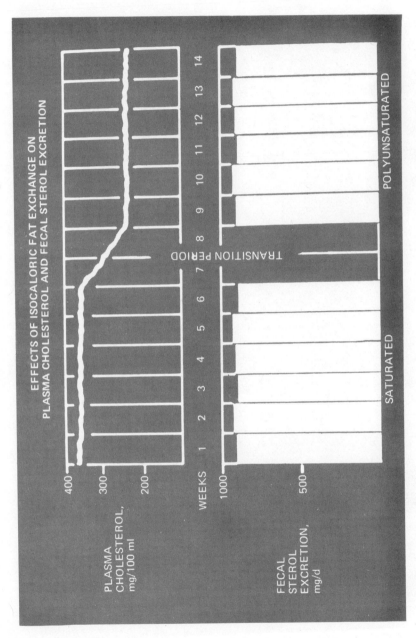

Fig. 4. When a polyunsaturated fat (corn oil) is isocalorically exchanged for a more saturated fat (butter) then plasma cholesterol decreases. In the experiment illustrated here total fecal cholesterol excretion did not increase correspondingly.

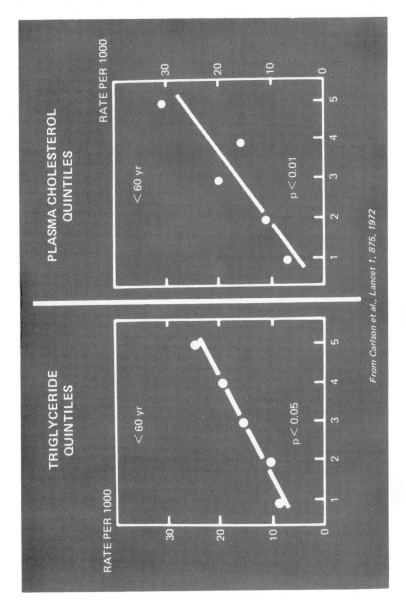

From Carlson et al., Lancet 1, 875, 1972

Fig. 5. Modification of Fig. 3 and Fig. 4, reference 7. In a 9-year prospective study of over 3000 Swedish men, the incidence of ischemic heart disease correlated linearly with plasma levels of triglyceride or cholesterol.

the men for plasma triglycerides on the left and plasma cholesterol
on the right. The numbers 1 through 5 refer to quintiles. That is,
all men are distributed from the 20% with lowest lipids to the 20%
with highest. It can be seen that the higher the triglyceride concentration the greater the risk of heart disease.

Fig. 6 illustrates the effect of alcohol upon serum triglycerides. When we (8) gave 150 cc of 44% (v/v) whiskey to several
men and followed their serum triglycerides for 12 hours thereafter,
we found the following: triglycerides rose slightly and then returned to baseline by 12 hours. When the men ingested 100 cc of
corn oil their triglycerides rose higher but also returned to normal
by 12 hours. However, when the fat and ethanol were drunk together
serum triglycerides increased over 300% and were still elevated 12
hours later. I would therefore recommend that patients with hypertriglyceridemia restrict their use of alcohol and that physicians
measuring plasma lipids should pay special attention to their patients foregoing a few cocktails the evening before the test.

IV. OBESITY

We have recently studied (9) the cholesterol metabolism of 8
very obese patients. Their mean cholesterol turnover was twice
that of comparable lean patients (Fig. 7). These findings were
confirmed by long-term radioisotopic cholesterol turnover studies.
The production rates were again twice those of normal weighted patients. We also found a large increase in the slowly turning-over
pool of body cholesterol. In further studies of human adipose tissue I have found that all of this expanded body pool of cholesterol
can be accounted for by the adipose tissue cholesterol content.
The amount of cholesterol stored in each fat cell or adipocyte is
dependent on the size of the cell. In other words the more triglyceride, the more cholesterol. Indeed, 90% of the cell cholesterol
is recovered in the intracellular oil droplet and not with membra-
nes (10).

These findings explain the increased body cholesterol storage
in obesity but what of the accelerated cholesterol synthesis? To
answer this question we obtained adipose tissue from obese patients
and measured the incorporation of radioactive glucose into cholesterol. The results showed very little cholesterol synthesis under a
wide variety of conditions. These included addition of insulin to
the medium, and varying the diets or reducing the patients' weights.

When these in vitro results are compared with the synthesis
rates obtained by sterol balance methods in vivo, the adipocytes
synthesized less than 1 mg of cholesterol per kg fat per day whereas the obese patients made over 20 mg cholesterol per kg excess
weight per day. We are now actively investigating causes for excessive cholesterol synthesis in obesity other than local adipose
tissue synthesis.

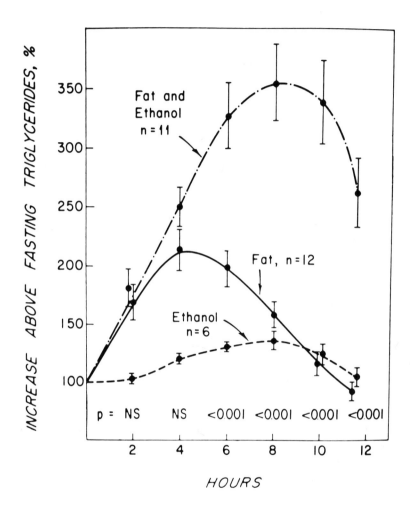

Fig. 6. From Fig. 1, reference 8. Serum triglyceride rise as percent of control after fat and ethanol, singly and in combination.

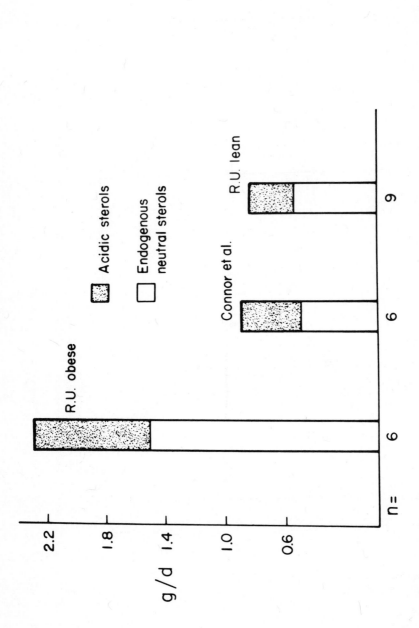

Fig. 7. The daily cholesterol turnover in 6 obese patients compared to 6 normals (ref. 3) and 9 hyperlipidemic but lean patients on similar diets (ref. 5).

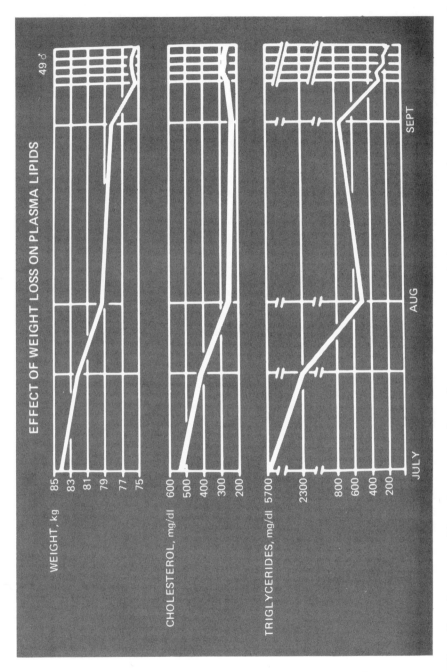

Fig. 8. Corresponding decreases in weight and plasma lipids of a 49-year-old man over a $2\frac{1}{2}$ month period.

There is another lipid abnormality associated with obesity, namely, hypertriglyceridemia. Overeating raises plasma triglycerides, sometimes so markedly that in the patient illustrated in Fig. 8, triglyceride levels reached 5700 mg% and cholesterol was over 500 mg%. By a relatively minor reduction of calories, his weight fell 2 kg and lipid concentrations halved. With further weight loss over the next 3 months, lipid levels practically normalized. This same patient had hard cutaneous xanthomata present for over 7 years. These disappeared completely after 3 months of weight reduction and have not returned during the past 2 years.

SUMMARY

Although I have discussed the role of dietary cholesterol, fat, alcohol and calories on serum lipids, we are primarily interested in lipids because they are related to atherosclerosis. In America, this disease alone accounts for over half of all deaths each year. We must, however, balance the urgency of the problem with the sober scientific reality that we still do not know how diet affects this disease in man nor do we know what the most ideal diet should be for the prevention or regression of the atherosclerotic plaque.

REFERENCES

1. Mattson, F.H., Erickson, B.A. and Kligman, A.M.
   Amer. J. Clin. Nutr. 25: 589, 1972.
2. Quintao, E., Grundy, S.M. and Ahrens, E.H., Jr.
   J. Lipid Res. 12: 233, 1971.
3. Connor, W.E., Witiak, D.T., Stone, D.B. and Armstrong, M.L.
   J. Clin. Invest. 48: 1363, 1969.
4. Moore, R.B., Anderson, J.T., Taylor, H.L., Keys, A.
   and Franz, I.D., Jr.
   J. Clin. Invest. 47: 1517, 1968.
5. Grundy, S.M. and Ahrens, E.H., Jr.
   J. Clin. Invest. 49: 1135, 1970.
6. Avigan, J. and Steinberg, D.
   J. Clin. Invest. 44: 1845, 1965.
7. Carlson, L.A. and Böttiger, L.E.
   Lancet 1: 865, 1972.
8. Wilson, D.E., Schreibman, P.H., Brewster, A.C. and Arky, R.A.
   J. Lab. Clin. Med. 75: 264, 1970.
9. Nestel, P.J., Schreibman, P.H. and Ahrens, E.H., Jr.
   J. Clin. Invest. 52: 2389, 1973.
10. Schreibman, P.H.
    Clin. Res. 21: 638a, 1973.

OUTLINES OF DIETARY PREVENTION OF ATHEROSCLEROSIS

R. ANGELICO

Istituto Superiore di Sanità, Rome, Italy

The attention of nutritionists and physicians given to the possibility of contributing, by the diet, to the prevention of atherosclerosis and its consequences, has arisen from two aspects of respective information:

- that deriving from studies on experimental atherosclerosis;
- and that deriving from anatomopathological, clinical, epidemiological and experimental studies carried out on populations of different countries.

It has been shown by research on experimental atherosclerosis (1,2) that, by confluence of various exogenous and endogenous factors, a high fat, high cholesterol diet represents the principal means for obtaining hypercholesterolemia, lipid infiltrations and atheromatous damage to the arterial walls.

These lesions are partly reversible and may regress together with hypercholesterolemia if the atherogenic diet is replaced by a diet with a normal lipid content.

Working on rats, an animal species considered very resistant, we have ourselves (3) observed that already after two months of treatment with hyperlipid diets integrated with cholesterol, a conspicuous increase of the lipid and cholesterol content of the liver serum and a significant increase of the cholesterol esters fraction of the aortic walls was observed. These changes reached even higher values when the treatment was continued, but regressed completely when the animals were reverted to a normal diet.

The anatomopathological, clinical, epidemiological and experimental findings on man (4,5,6,7,8,9), even if not completely conclusive, and often contradictory, have substantially demonstrated a number of objective facts, illustrated by the speakers of this course. We will try to enumerate them in their logical sequence:

- in the atheromatous plaques of the walls of the large and medium arteries an accumulation of lipid material has been noticed, especially that of cholesterol;

- these alterations are generally connected with an increase of the concentrations of lipids or some fractions in blood;

- populations with a diet low in calories, total lipids, saturated fats, cholesterol and rich in starch, do generally present moderate lipid blood levels;

- apart from a few exceptions, in the blood of populations habitually feeding on diets excessive in calories, in relations to energy expenditure, high in total fats, saturated fats, cholesterol and sugars, frequently higher levels of total lipids, cholesterol and often triglycerides are found;

- populations which have enriched totally or partially their diet, often show higher lipid levels than in the past;

- the contrary has been observed in populations which were obliged to reduce their food consumption to a minimum, as have been noted in war and postwar conditions;

- high blood lipid levels induced by a diet (and especially levels higher than 260 mg % ml of cholesterol) are, in some way, involved in the pathogenesis of atherosclerosis and its consequences, and are considered, together with hypertension and excessive cigarette smoking, the main risk factors, while minor factors, but not less important, are inherited and ambiental factors, diabetes, obesity, alteration of blood coagulation, lack of exercise, psycho-social tensions, etc.;

- suitable changes of dietary habits, especially of diets, consisting in reduction of total calories, fats and cholesterol, substitution of saturated with unsaturated fats, if applied early enough, can favourably influence abnormal lipid pictures and reduce morbidity and mortality from atherosclerosis and its consequences (primary prevention), and prevent the repetition and aggravation of pathological events (secondary prevention).

Considering these concepts valid, we can try to critically examin how the various dietary components may influence the levels of blood lipids, and how to intervene consequently in this preventive action.

CALORIE INTAKE

Epidemiology teaches us that a "rich" diet is involved in pathogenesis and ethiology of cardiovascular diseases and contributes to the development of obesity, hypertriglyceridemia, hyperglycemia, hyperuricemia, all implicated as risk factors.

A correction of these biochemical parameters by arranging the total caloric intake in order to reach and maintain an ideal body weight, is considered to be a reasonable way in constituting a preventive regimen.

In some countries the different incidence of coronary diseases seems to depend more on the total calorie intake, than on specific factors. Yet the effect is not well defined, it seems to depend on energy expenditure and also on individual differences in food utilization. Weight reduction frequently lowers elevated serum lipids.

TOTAL FAT INTAKE

The quantity of total fats in the diet seems to have a great influence on blood lipid levels. Populations with high fat diets, generally present high levels of serum cholesterol; populations with poor lipid diets have low levels of cholesterolemia. Anyway it seems that, at similar lipid intake, considerable individual variations exist.

According to KEYS and WHITE, populations with fat intakes approximately 40% of the total calories have high coronary death rates; population with total fat intakes below 20% of the total calories have low death rates; populations with intermediate fat intake have intermediate death rates (10).

QUALITY OF DIETARY FATS

KEYS (11) has emphasized how the proportion of dietetic calories coming from saturated fatty acids has a direct effect upon the cholesterol levels in the plasma. The saturated fatty acids seem to be twice as effective in increasing the serum cholesterol levels than as the polyunsaturated acids are in reducing them; monounsaturated fatty acids seem to have a negligible effect.

It should be noted, as to polyunsaturated fatty acids, whose crucial importance in the synthesis of prostaglandines is well known, that the Eskimos, who are the only nation on Earth having a diet made up, in its lipid part, exclusively of unsaturated fats, have the lowest levels of blood cholesterol and a very rare incidence of coronary diseases (12).

The different effect of dietary fats on serum cholesterol seems to depend, apart of on the degree of fatty acids saturation, also on the high content of essential fatty acids, or on the presence of trace elements as the phytosterols in vegetal oils, or on the length of the chain. Lauric acid (C 12), miristic acid (C 14), and palmitic acid (C 16) are capable of increasing serum cholesterol more than stearic acid (of 18 carbon atoms), which may, moreover, induce hypertriglyceridemia (13).

The problem therefore should be seen more correctly in these terms, rather than as a question of animal and plant fats. In fact, most animal fats are rich in saturated fatty acids, but some, as those of fishes, have a high degree of unsaturation; on the contrary, most vegetal oils are rich in unsaturated fats, although some rich in saturated fatty acids exist.

It should be remembered how the composition of animal fats can vary according to the feeding pattern and the season, while the composition of vegetal fats may vary according to production methods. Modifications of their capacity of influencing cholesterol levels may also derive from the way food is prepared and heated, which fact may induce polymerization and the production of toxic products, from industrial procedures of hydrogenation with saturation, changes of the double link positions, formation of "trans" forms, conjugations, etc.

The conclusion however is, that the ratio between saturated and polyunsaturated fatty acids in diet is remarkably correlated to the levels of blood cholesterol (14); even if recently there have been discordant opinions on the subject.

For example, in a recent article in the American Journal of Clinical Nutrition, Reiser (15) critically sustains that the idea of a hypercholestemic action of saturated fatty acids does derive, rather than from a direct demonstration, from the hypocholesterolemic effect of unsaturated fatty acids. The author finds some conclusions on the subject as arbitrary and due to experimental errors or mistakes in the interpretation of results.

We therefore think that a clarification of perplexities is necessary in order to evaluate the validity of dietetic prescriptions formed according to the predominant opinion valid so far.

Another controversal argument is the importance given by CONNOR (16) to the amount of dietary cholesterol as effective in regulating blood cholesterol levels. This effect is less evident in humans than in animals fed experimental diets (17).

According to some authors, the dietetic cholesterol is absolutely the most important factor in establishing the levels of blood cholesterol, according to others, it is responsible only for 60-80% of the latter. According to KEYS (18), exogenous cholesterol increases the serum levels in proportion to the square-root of its concentration in the diet.

It must be remembered that the daily intake of cholesterol in an average medium diet may vary from 200 to 800 mg; while the endogenous synthesis can supply daily approximately 2000 mg or even more.

A partial explanation of the correlation, not always confirmed, between dietary and blood cholesterol can be given by the finding that endogenous synthesis of cholesterol can be inhibited by the excessive intake of dietetic cholesterol through a feedback mechanism.

In preventive diets a daily intake lower than 300 mg is advisable, although other authors find it necessary to impose stronger restrictions (down to 100 mg), which are practically difficult to realize.

QUANTITY AND QUALITY OF DIETARY CARBOHYDRATES

The quantitative aspect is identical with the total caloric intake already mentioned.

The importance of dietetic carbohydrates in influencing blood levels of lipids and consequently in the pathogenesis of atherosclerosis has been shown by:

- the evidence, obtained by Ahrens (19), of the existence of a carbohydrate induced hypertriglyceridemia;

- the possibility, shown by McDonald (20), of provoking hypertriglyceridemia, hypercholesterolemia, hyperglycerimia in normal subjects by intake of sucrose or fructose;

- the increase, reported by Yudkin (21) and other authors, of vascular diseases in population having substituted their traditional alimentary habits, based on cereals and vegetables, with larger consumption of simple sugars.

We have ourselves (22) been able to confirm the hypothesis that dietary carbohydrates, according to their type, may differently influence lipid metabolism. The presence of soluble carbohydrates in normolipidic diets caused an increase of the triglyceride levels of the liver and, at the same time, a very high increase of some enzymatic activities related to lipogenesis. With atherogenic, hyperlipidic diets integrated with cholesterol, the increase of cholesterol in the plasma, liver and aortic walls was higher in rats receiving glucose or sucrose, than in those receiving starch. As can be seen, the phenomenon is reproduced, although with different mechanisms, which will not be discussed here. Yet during this course we were shown different results, although obtained on other animal species.

This theory is however strongly criticized by Keys (23), who consider it absolutely not acceptable as well from the clinical and the epidemiological, as the theoretical and experimental points of view. In a recent paper the author reports the existence of populations having a high intake of sugar and fruit with low blood lipid levels and rare cardiovascular diseases. He underlines that generally a high intake of sugar is accompanied by a high intake of saturated fats and cholesterol as well as by excessive smoking and coffee drinking etc., which are also considered as important risk factors.

Biochemical information exists by which it can be shown that the different response to various dietary sugars may be interpreted by the diversity of metabolic pathways followed in the endogenous synthesis of lipids.

It however seems that individual variations are of noteworthy importance due also to a certain percentage of individuals who are particularly sensitive to some carbohydrates. Consequently the effects of the quantity and quality of dietary carbohydrates must be evaluated with extreme caution (since in some cases, the studies made are of short duration). Although the extremes to incriminate, in accordance with Yudkin, sugar do not exist, it seems not even possible to rigorously exclude that soluble carbohydrates may at least be considered additional factors to lipids in their effects on the blood lipid picture.

It seems therefore reasonable to suggest their limitation, giving more space to complex carbohydrates. Yet research should be extended to particular population groups (24).

This argument anyway draws attention to hypertriglyceridemia, associated or not with hypercholesterolemia, as a risk-factor of atherosclerosis. This fact, as though indirectly shown in studies by Framingham (25), has been confirmed by epidemiologic studies in Sweden. Recently Albrink (26) has reported about an indipendent risk-factor involved, by still unknown mechanisms, with some symptomatic manifestations of coronary disease.

Hypertriglycedemia is generally a primary phenomenon, indipendent from dietary introductions of carbohydrates. Nevertheless it can be increased by sugar consumption and be reduced when calorie and sugar intakes are restricted.

ALCOHOL

It has been noted that atherosclerosis and ischaemic heart disease are uncommon in alcoholized persons. This seems to be proved in some areas in France, where the alcohol consumption is very high. It is rather probable that the abnormal diet of alcoholics may play as great a role in the casual relationship as the alcohol

intake itself. An excessive alcohol intake may cause hypertriglyceridemia; in fact endogenous production of lipids, with a high
level of blood lipoproteins rich in triglycerides, is exaggerated
when the main caloric intake derives either from alcohol or from
carbohydrates (10).

DIETARY PROTEIN LEVEL

An adequate protein level does not effect the **serum cholesterol.**
Very little indeed is known about the relationship between dietary
protein intake, blood lipid levels and occurence of atherosclerosis.

Suppositions have been made that serum lipids might be influenced not only by fat and cholesterol but also by proteins: hyperlipidic
diets being also rich in animal proteins and an increase of these
proteins is by some author related to mortality caused by coronary
diseases.

A reduction of serum cholesterol and of the percentage of betalipoproteins is claimed, even with cholesterol present in the
diet, when the quantity of dietary proteins is less than 25 grams
per day. This hypocholesterolemia has been attributed to deficien-
ces of free methyl groups, methionin being probably the main limiting aminoacid in this effect.

Olson found more evident hypocholesterolemic effects in man by
supplying synthetic diets containing all the eight essential amino-
acids plus glutammate as the only source of non essential amino-
acids to provide the minimum nitrogen requirement.

There are contradictory opinions regarding experiments in which
an accumulation of serum cholesterol seems to have been obtained,
supplying dietary proteins low in sulphur, due to the inhibition
of the formation of bile acids conjugated with taurine. It thus
can clearly be seen how controversial this argument is.

MINERALS

Excess of sodium chloride is related to the incidence of hypertension considered an important risk-factor in vascular diseases
(29). The hypotensive diets based on fruit were, in fact, poor in
sodium and rich in potassium. A daily supply of salt not superior
to 5 g is advisable, this quantity may of course be varied according to the climate and to the physical activity.

A similar correlation seems to have been demonstrated in regard to cadmium (30), which can be found in abnormally high concentrations in kidneys of hypertensive subjects.

According to epidemiologic research by Schroeder (31), total
cardiovascular death rates are inversely related to the hardness
of drinking water: which fact would draw further attention to the

effects of other elements such as calcium, magnesium, carbonates, lead, sulfates, etc. (32).

Conversion of acetic acid into cholesterol in the liver is depressed by vanadium and iron, and increased by chromium and manganese.

Chromium deserves a special note, since it is considered as a potenciating factor of the insulin's action. Tissue chromium deficience together with a decreased carbohydrate tollerance, hyper-triglyceridemia and an increase in atherosclerosis have been noted particularly in economically advanced countries where large quantities of highly refined sugars are eaten. Unrefined sugars and complex carbohydrates contain enough chromium to cover these losses: and their protective action may thus be explained (33).

VITAMINS

To pay attention to nicotinic acid, which at high doses (1 to 6 g per day) significantly reduces blood levels of cholesterol by enzymatic mechanisms at the level of synthesis in the liver and by the conversion of bile acids, would mean to displace the question into a pharmacological basis, which is not our intention nor competence.

The same approach is true for vitamin A: the hypocholesterol-emic action of vitamin A has been shown after long treatments with 100,000 I.U. per day.

As for vitamin B_6, without considering some experimental data, there seems to be no elements regarding its importance as an athero-genous factor in man (10).

It is suggested that vitamin E should be present in diets rich in polyunsaturated fatty acids, advisable for hypercholesterolemic individuals, due to its antioxidative action capable of preventing the formation of free radicals in relation to some theories on aging. A daily supply of large amounts of unsaturated fatty acids, especially linoleic acid, increases the requirement for vitamin. However generally food of vegetal origin which contains polyunsaturated fatty acids contains also vitamin E, even if small amounts are found in refined aliments. Even if toxicological limitations do not exist, it seems not justifiable to promote an excessive intake of products containing vitamin E, as happens in some countries (34-35).

Regarding witamin C we cannot not remember the recent research of Czechoslovak Authors, who have shown that with a chronic lack of this vitamin there is an increase of serum cholesterol and betalipo-proteins due to a reduction of the hepatic conversion of cholesterol in bile acids, postulating a possible role of vitamin C deficiency in the pathogenesis of metabolic lesions which are at the base of atherosclerosis, and suggesting a possible use of this vitamin for integrating preventive dietary treatments (36).

To conclude, the presence of vitamins is a general nutritional need, without any specific indications.

DIETARY FIBER

Dietary fiber has been defined as the skeletal remains of plant cells, that are resistant to hydrolysis by the enzymes of men. The possible role of these unavailable carbohydrates as cellulose, lignine, pentosans, uronic acids and of pectines against hyperlipemia and ischemic heart disease has been noticed in the low blood cholesterol levels of vegetarian people and of populations consuming natural starchy carbohydrates.

It is suggested that dietary fiber sequestrates bile acids decreasing the reabsorption of bile salts, increasing fecal excretion and reducing hyperlipidemia (37).

MEAL FREQUENCY

Attention has been called from experimental research made by American Authors (38) - which we ourselves (39) have only partially been able to confirm - upon the possibility that the feeding frequency may influence the utilization of the diet even indipendently of its quantity and qualitative composition.

According to Fabry (40), even in man, the consumption of all the daily diet into 3 meals increases the body weight and levels of serum lipids, particularly of cholesterol. This does not happen if the same quantity of food is eaten in more meals (5 or 6).

It cannot be excluded that deviding the food intake into a higher number of meals, may be of a certain validity if applied to the dietary prevention of atherosclerosis.

Let us now try to draw some conclusions and give some general dietary indications still remaining in a general orientation of the discussion which others can transform better than ourselves, into practical application.

According to recommendations of the American Heart Association (41), integrated with the opinion of Italian nutritionists (42-43), and what may derive from the (present review, it may by attempted to formulate a dietetic) prevention scheme of atherosclerosis in the following manner summarized in Table I:

1) adjust the total calorie supply to the energy need, in order to achieve and maintain invaried as far as possible, the optimal body weight;

Table I. Dietary scheme in atherosclerosis prevention

1) TOTAL CALORIE INTAKE	RELATED TO ENERGY EXPENDITURE
2) TOTAL FAT INTAKE	NOT OVER 30% OF TOTAL CALORIES
3) SATURATED FAT INTAKE	NOT OVER 10% OF TOTAL CALORIES
	(isocaloric quantities of saturated, mono-and polyunsaturated)
4) CHOLESTEROL INTAKE	NOT MORE THAN 300 mg PER DAY
5) CARBOHYDRATE INTAKE	RELATED TO ENERGY EXPENDITURE
	(limiting sugars·and using with preference starch)
6) PROTEIN INTAKE IN THE RANGE OF NEED, ADEQUATE INTAKE OF MINERALS AND VITAMINS, MODERATE ALCOHOL INTAKE	
7) SALT INTAKE MAX. 5 grams PER DAY	
8) SUBDIVISION OF THE TOTAL FOOD INTAKE INTO A HIGH NUMBER OF DAILY MEALS (over 5)	

2) reduce the total dietary fat to no more than 30% of the total calories (which fact will limit the total calories, will reduce avoid postprandial hyperlipemia and its possible adverse effects on blood coagulation, and reduce the large absorption of cholesterol due to an excess in dietary fat);

3) reduce the intake of saturated fatty acids to no more than 10% of the total calories, with a commensurate increase of unsaturated fatty acids. Isocaloric quantities of saturated, monounsaturated and polyunsaturated fats can be recommended. (In practice this means the elimination of animal lipids, lard, butter, fat cheese etc., highly hydrogenized margarine, high fat meat, cream and to enhance the intake of fish, lean meat, skim milk, soft margarines, cottagecheese, olive and seed oil, excluding palm and cocconut oil, rich in saturated fats);

4) restrict the dietary cholesterol to no morethan 300 mg per day, excluding food containing high quantities of it, as egg-yolk, entrails, and not forgetting that meat contains approx. 90 mg cholesterol in 100 g;

5) regulate the carbohydrate and alcohol intake in relation to the energy expenditure, limiting sugars and prefering instead complex carbohydrates present in cereals and vegetables.

6) mantain the protein intake in the range of the requirement, with a correct balance between animal and vegetal proteins, and assure an adequate intake of vitamins and minerals;

7) limit salt intake to not more than 5 g per day;

8) tend to consume the total daily food intake in as many meals as possible.

In order to put into practice with efficiency the above mentioned dietary recommendations, attention should be paid to the following necessities:

- to introduce their application at an early stage (changes of food habits are easier and better during childhood and youth), and once applied they should be continuously respected in order to become life rules;

- to keep in mind that any kind of dietary restriction or food habit changes must be accepted consciously, without causing neither preoccupation nor anxiety, or clamorous breakings with rooted traditions, or domestic difficulties and must be undertaken with suitables recepies to avoid monotonous and untasty diets;

- to avoid that the dietary advice should compromise the intake of essential nutrients causing deficiencies and loss of equilibrium;

- to avoid that social - economic conditions of populations induce bad alimentary habits;

- to obtain through an intensification of dietary surveys a better knowledge of the real nutritional conditions of populations;

- to develop nutritional educational programs in order to develop good habits and knowledge of the real value of food-stuffs and the influence that cooking may have on them;

- to provide in markets modified and ordinary foods useful for the purpose, reasonable priced and appropriately labeled, avoiding an inadequate and excessive advertising. As can be seen the problem glides over to production, preparation, preservation and marketing systems. Agricolture and Food Industry, in the field of common or special foodstuffs, can efficiently cooperate to this end.

     The preventive dietary rules above mentioned should be applied on a large scale with the so called "privileged" groups of the population, in which epidemiology reveals a higher level of atherosclerotic diseases. Yet an early application is absolutely necessary, together with healthy life habits in those apparently healthy individuals considered in "special risk categories" because of hereditary or environmental reasons. It is therefore necessary to identify these subjects within the whole population. This can be obtained, as the first of any prevention action, by anamnestic investigation, by clinical controls of the health conditions of the populations, particularly by the knowledge of their lipid profile, i.e. of the haematochemical parameters, not limited to the cholesterolemia control only, but extended to the total lipid pattern, to lipemia, triglyceridemia, quantitative determination of the blood lipoprotein families, and, last but not least, other auxiliary tests (43). If these controls, replicated more than once with appropriate techniques, indicate the existence of nonaccidental abnormalities, the selection and classification of individuals into types, although the latter may be subject to discussion, can be carried out (44,45,46).

     The classification into different types of human hyperlipoproteinaemias was the main argument of a Course which was held, last year, in this same Institute and before that in Milan (47). It is performed in our country by the Italian Society of Atherosclerosis Studies, and its President, Prof. Paoletti. The typing permits the differential diagnosis of the various forms on a genetic basis, it gives the possibility of identifying other alterations which may induce atherosclerosis and to identify action mechanisms, and allows adequate and specific treatments. We cannot, today, be satisfied with overall solutions.

Table II. DIET FOR TYPE II (hyperbetalipoproteinaemia with
increase of cholesterol and in
some cases of triglycerides (II b))

CALORIES	NOT RESTRICTED (in the range of the need)
PROTEINS	NOT LIMITED (1 g/Kg body weight - 10-20% total cal.)
LIPIDS	25% OF TOTAL CALORIES (proportionally increased in II b) (saturated limited - P/S = 1,8-2,8)
CHOLESTEROL	RESTRICTED (100-200 mg per day; from meat only)
CARBOHYDRATES	NOT RESTRICTED (65% of total calories, limited to 40% in II b)
ALCOHOL	TO BE USED WITH DISCRETION

Table III. DIET FOR TYPE IV   (hyperprebetalipoproteinaemia with
                                increase of endogenous triglycerides)

CALORIES   CONTROLLED

                            (to achieve and mantain the "optimal"
                             body weight)

PROTEINS   NOT LIMITED

                            (1 g/Kg body weight)

LIPIDS   NOT LIMITED

                            (preference to polyunsaturated)

CHOLESTEROL   MODERATELY REDUCED

                            (300-500 mg per day)

CARBOHYDRATES   CONTROLLED

                            (max. 40% of total calories;
                             without sweets)

ALCOHOL   LIMITED

                            (in any case in substitution of
                             carbohydrates)

As shown in Table II and III (based on recommendations of N.I.H.), the dietary menagement will be different for the two most frequent types of hyperlipoproteinaemias (II and IV) in which the abnormality, single or predominant, is hypercholesterolemia in the first and hypertriglyceridemia in the second case (48).

In conclusion we would like to point out that, according to our points of view, while the diet is one of the most valid arms of prevention, it is only one of the various components in the genesis and prevention of diseases of multifactorial ethiology.

The more this will be kept in mind, the more are the possibilities of success.

Today it is frequently said that "we are what we eat", but the clinical nutritionist must also, with conscious humility, as says Brock (49) (in the introduction to his chapter on the general orientation of dietology) take into consideration that, if this is true, it is also true that "we are what we are born", yet it goes without discussion that "we also are what our environment allows our genotype to become".

REFERENCES

1. Costantinides, P.
   Experimental Atherosclerosis.
   Elsevier, Amsterdam, 1965.
2. Armstrong, M.L., Warner, E.D. and Connor, W.E.
   Regression of coronary atheromatosis in Rhesus monkeys.
   Circulation Research, 27: 59, 1970.
3. Angelico, R., Casparrini, G., Cavina, G. and Moretta, L.
   Effetti della somministrazione continua o discontinua di
   una dieta "aterogena" sulla composizione lipidica di siero,
   fegato, e aorta di ratto.
   Ann. Ist. Sup. Sanità, 4: 234, 1968.
4. Stamler, J.
   Acute Myocardial Infarction - Progress in primary prevention.
   Brit. Heart Journal, Suppl. 33: 145, 1971.
5. Epstein, F.M.
   Epidemiologic aspects of atherosclerosis.
   Atheroscl. 14: 1, 1971.
6. Strong, J.K., Eggen, D.A., Oalmann, M.C. and Tracy, R.E.
   Pathology and epidemiology of atherosclerosis.
   Journ. Am. Diet. Assoc. 62: 262, 1973.

7. Turpeinen, O., Miettinen, M., Karvonen, M.J., Roine, P.,
   Perkarinen, M., Lehtosuo, E.J. and Alivirta, P.:
   Dietary prevention of coronary heart disease: long term
   experiment.
   Am. J. Clin. Nutr. 21:, 255, 1968.
8. Wen, C. and Gershoff, S.N.:
   Changes in serum cholesterol and coronary heart disease
   mortality associated with changes in the postwar Japanese diet.
   Am. J. Clin. Nutr. 26: 616, 1973.
9. Report of Inter-Society Commission for heart Disease Resources.
   Primary prevention of atherosclerosis diseases.
   Circulation, 12: 55, 1970.
10. Friedman, G.J.:
    Nutrition in relation to atherosclerosis, in: Wohl M.G.,
    Goodharth R.S. - Modern Nutrition in Health and Disease.
    IV Ed., Lea a. Febiger, Philadelphia, 1968, chapt. 29B.
11. Keys, A.:
    Coronary heart disease in seven countries.
    Circulation, Suppl. 41: 1, 1970.
12. Banc, H.O., Dyerberg, J. and Brondum Nielsen, A.:
    Plasma lipid and lipoprotein pattern in Greenlandic West
    Coast Eskimos.
    Lancet, 1: 1143, 1971.
13. Grande, F., Anderson, J.T. and Keys, A.:
    Diets of different fatty acid composition producing
    identical serum cholesterol levels in man.
    Am. J. Clin. Nutr. 25: 53, 1972.
14. Anderson, J.T., Grande, F. and Keys, A.:
    Cholesterol-lowering diets.
    Journ. Am. Diet. Assoc. 62: 133, 1973.
15. Reiser, R.:
    Saturated fat in the diet and serum cholesterol concentration:
    a critical examination of the literature.
    Am. J. Clin. Nutr., 26: 524, 1973.
16. Mattson, F.H., Erickson, B.A. and Kligman, A.M.:
    Effect of dietary cholesterol on serum cholesterol in man.
    Am. J. Clin. Nutr. 25: 589, 1972.
17. Connor, W.E., Hodges, R.E. and Bleiler, R.A.:
    The serum lipids in men receiving high cholesterol and
    free cholesterol-free diets.
    J. Clin. Invest. 40: 894, 1961.
18. Fetcher, E.S., Foster, N., Anderson, J.T., Grande, F. and
    Keys, A.: Quantitative estimation of diet control serum
    cholesterol.
    Am. J. of Clin. Nutr. 20: 475, 1967.
19. Ahrens, E.H. Jr., Hirsch, J., Oette, K., Fabquhar, J.W. and
    Stein, Y.: Carbohydrate-induced and fat-induced lipemia.
    Trans. Assoc. Am. Physicians, 74: 134, 1961.

20. Macdonald, I.:
    Relationship between dietary carbohydrates and lipid
    metabolism. Nutritio et Dieta.
    Symposium Bibl. 15: 129, 1970.
21. Yudkin, J.:
    Dietary fat and dietary sugar in relation to ischaemic
    heart disease and diabetes.
    Lancet ii: 4, 1964.
22. Angelico, R., Moretta, L., Improta, G. and Ialongo, P.:
    Effects of dietary carbohydrates on body lipid composition
    and on some enzymatic activities in the rat.
    Nutr. Metabol. 12: 179, 1970.
23. Keys, A.:
    Sucrose in the diet and coronary heart disease.
    Atherosclerosis, 14: 193, 1971.
24. Walker, A.R.P.:
    Sugar intake and coronary heart disease.
    Atherosclerosis, 14: 137, 1971.
25. Kannel, W.B., Castelli, W.P., Gordon, T. and McNamara, P.M.:
    Serum cholesterol, lipoproteins and the risk of coronary
    heart disease. The Framingham Study.
    Ann. Int. Med. 74: 1, 1971.
26. Carlson, L.A. and Bottiger, L.E.:
    Ischaemic heart disease in relation to fasting values of
    plasma triglycerides and cholesterol.
    Stockolm Prospective Study - Lancet 1:, 865, 1972.
27. Albrink, M.J.:
    Triglyceridemia.
    J. Am. Diet. Assoc., 62: 626, 1973.
28. Olson, R.E., Milton, Z.N., Nittka, J. and Eagles, J.A.:
    Effect of amino acid diets upon serum lipids in man.
    Am. J. Clin. Nutr. 23: 1614, 1970.
29. Perry, H.M.:
    Minerals in cardiovascular disease.
    Am. J. Diet. Assoc., 62: 631, 1973.
30. Schroeder, H.A.:
    Cadmium as a factor in hypertension.
    J. Chron. Dis. 18: 647, 1965.
31. Schroeder, H.A.:
    Relations between hardness of water and death rates from
    certain chronic and degenerative diseases in the U.S.
    J. Chron. Dis. 12: 586, 1960.
32. Morris, J.N., Crawford, M.D. and Heady, J.A.:
    Hardness of local water supplies and mortality from
    cardiovascular disease in the county boroughs of
    England and Wales.
    Lancet 1: 860, 1961.

33. Schroeder, M.A.:
    The role of chromium in mammalian nutrition.
    Am. J. Clin. Nutr. 21: 230, 1968.
34. Christiansen, M.M. and Wilcox, E.B.:
    Dietary polyunsaturates and serum alphatocopherol in adults.
    J. Am. Diet. Ass. 63: 138, 1973.
35. Hodges, R.E.:
    Vitamin E and coronary heart disease.
    J. Am. Diet. Ass. 63: 638, 1973.
36. Ginter, E.:
    The role of ascorbic acid in cholesterol metabolism.
    Vydav. Slov. Acad. Vied, Bratislava, 1970.
37. Trowell, H.:
    Ischemic heart disease and dietary fiber.
    Am. J. Clin. Nutr. 25: 926, 1972.
38. Cohn, C., Joseph, D. and Allweiss, M.D.:
    Studies on the effects of feeding frequency and dietary
    composition on fat deposition.
    Ann. N.Y. Acad. of Sc. 131: 507, 1965.
39. Angelico, R., Ferro-Luzzi, A., Frasca, M.A., Mariani, A.,
    Migliaccio, P.A. and Moretta, L.:
    Ricerche sui rapporti fra ritmo di assunzione e utilizzazione
    nutritiva della dieta.
    Quaderni Nutrizione, 27: 233, 1967.
40. Fabry, P., Fodor, J., Geizerova, H., Heil, Z.,
    Balcarova, O. and Zwolankova, K.:
    Meal frequency and ischaemic heart disease.
    Lancet ii: 190, 1968.
41. Mueller, J.F.:
    A dietary approach to coronary artery disease.
    J. Am. Diet. Assoc. 62: 613, 1973.
42. Mancini, M., Moro, C.O., Cuzzupoli, M., Di Marino, L. and
    Caputo, V.:
    La dieta nell'arteriosclerosi umana.
    Quad. Nutriz. 28: 6, 1968.
43. Fidanza, F.:
    Nutrition and Cardiovascular Disease. Secondary prevention
    and prospective epidemiological studies.
    Plen. lecture, Proc. Intern. Congr. Dietetics, Hannover, 1973.
44. Kannel, W.B.:
    Lipid profile and the potential coronary victim.
    Am. J. Clin. Nutr. 24: 1074, 1971.
45. Fredrickson, D.S., Levy, R.I. and Lees, R.S.:
    Fat transport in lipoproteins and integrated approach
    to mechanisms and disorders.
    New Engl. J. Med. 276: 34, 94, 148, 215, 273, 1967.

46. Levy, R.I., Bonnel, M. and Ernst, N.D.:
    Dietary menagement of hyperlipoproteinemia.
    J. Am. Diet. Assoc. 58: 406, 1971.
47. Classification of Hyperlipidaemias and hyperlipoproteinemias.
    Bull. Wld. Hlth Org. 43: 891, 1970.
48. Fumagalli, R., Ricci, G. and Gorini, S.:
    Human hyperlipoproteinemias - Principles and Methods -
    Proceedings of the Postgraduate Courses held in Milan, 1971
    and in Rome, 1972.
    Plenum Press, New York, London, 1973.
49. Angelico, R.:
    Lineamenti dietetici nelle iperlipoproteinemie primitive.
    Clin. Dietol. 1: 1974.
    In press.
50. Davidson, S., Passmore, R. and Brock, J.F.:
    Human Nutrition and Dietetics.
    V Ed. Churchill Livingstone, Edinburgh and London, 1972, p.307.

THE INFLUENCE OF DIETARY FATS ON HYPERCOAGULATION AND THROMBOSIS

JAMES M. IACONO

Lipid Nutrition Laboratory, Nutrition Institute, ARS
U.S. Department of Agriculture
Beltsville, Maryland 20705 USA

A distinct impression is emerging from the literature that nutrition plays an important role in haemostasis and thrombosis. Although present knowledge is sketchy and newer information is still needed to place nutritional-thrombotic interrelationships on a firm foundation, recent literature shows that dietary fats alter platelet function and that this might occur as a consequence of alterations of platelet lipids. Thus far, feeding studies in man and animals have shown alterations in platelet factor 3 (PF-3), platelet aggregation, and platelet lipids.

One of the earliest reported studies implicating nutrition as an environmental factor adversely affecting the clotting mechanism was that of Thomas and Hartroft (33). They were able to induce thrombosis in rats spontaneously by feeding a diet rich in saturated fat and cholesterol with the addition of thiouracil and cholic acid. Hartroft and O'Neal (5) found that the addition of cocoa butter or butter produced thrombi located to a great extent in the cardiac cavities and coronary arteries while plant oils such as cottonseed or corn oil protected the animals from these harmful effects. Similar observations have been made by other investigators in rats (4,17,19), rabbits (21), and pigs (15,16) by using various means to produce thrombus formation. A typical example of results obtained in rats is shown in Fig. 1. Of the many studies reported in animals, Renaud and Gautheron (22) conclude that the high saturated fat diet appears to "predispose to thrombosis while triggering agents such as ADP, endotoxin, or epinephrine most likely determine the location of the thrombi, whether it be in veins, the cardiac cavity or in arteries".

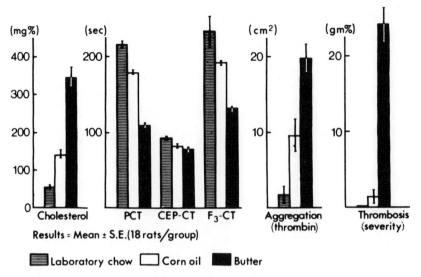

Fig. 1.   Influence of feeding various diets to rats for 10 weeks
on cholesterolemia, coagulation, platelet aggregation, and on
severity of thrombosis initiated by S. typhosa lipopolysaccharide
(0.3 mg/Kg).   PCT- plasma clotting time; CEP-CT - cephalin clotting time; F_3-CT - factor 3 clotting time;   (Courtesy of S. Renaud
and F. Lecompte, Circulat. Res. 37: 1003, 1970).

    What can we conclude from recent literature in regard to pla-
telet function and platelet lipid composition, and to what extent
can we assume that they have integrated functions after a given
diet?

    The need for PF-3 in blood coagulation is well established.
PF-3, a phospholipid, or a combination of phospholipids of platelets has been shown to be necessary in the clotting sequence.   In
in vitro studies, the most potent phospholipid in the coagulation
reaction has been shown to be phosphatidylserine (PS) (12,27,32),
acting as a single phospholipid or in combination with other phospholipids.   In his discussion of PF-3, Marcus (13) showed that this
factor most likely functions optimally in coagulation as a lipoprotein complex.   More recently, Renaud and Gautheron (22) made further progress in clarifying the role of phospholipids in coagulation.   They showed that when PS was extracted from platelets and
properly dispersed in an in vitro medium by sonication that the
activity of a given amount of the PS could completely replace PF-3
activity of the PS in its native form.

    It appears that PF-3 activity is dependent on the type of fat-
ty acids present in PS or PS + phosphatidylinositol (PI).   In feeding studies in rats (2), the ratio of stearic acid to linoleic acid
was closely correlated with experimental thrombosis, stearic acid

being the thrombogenic fatty acid of the diet and linoleic acid
counteracting the effect of stearic acid (Fig. 2). Analysis of
the platelet lipids of these rats also revealed a correlation between the PF-3 activity of the blood and the dietary modification
of the fatty acids of PS or PS + PI. Changes that occurred in
these phospholipids were an increase in stearic and oleic acids
and a decrease in polyunsaturated fatty acids when a saturated fat
was fed. The changes in the clotting activity appeared to be unrelated to the relative percentage of PS or PS + PI in platelets
since only slight changes were noted in the amounts of these phospholipids in platelets after various dietary fats were fed. The

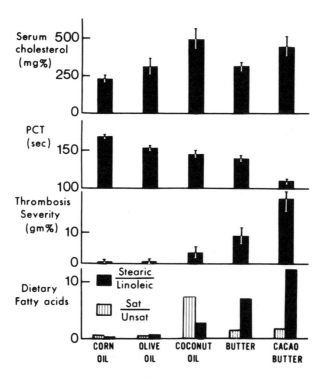

Results = Mean ± S.E. (15 to 24 determinations/group)

Fig. 2. Thrombogenic and cholesterolemic effects of dietary fatty
acids in rat. In addition to the usual ingredients, the diets contained either butter alone (38%) or butter (10%) added to 24% of
one of the fats listed in the figure. The ratios stearic/linoleic
acid or saturated/unsaturated fatty acids of the dietary fat combinations are reported in the figure, for each group. PCT - plasma clotting time. (Courtesy of P. Gautheron and S. Renaud, Thromb.
Res. 1, 353, 1972).

role of dietary fat on platelet lipid composition has been an area
that has provoked considerable interest. It has been shown that
changes in dietary fats cause the phospholipids of platelets to
undergo changes in composition of their fatty acids and even cause
changes in the relative distribution of the phospholipid classes.
Dietary studies in man as they relate to changes in the lipids of
platelets are now appearing in the literature. Nordöy and Rödset
(18) showed that soybean oil fed at 40% of calories for 21 days in
man gave significant increases in linoleic acid of choline, ethanolamine, and serine phosphoglucerides. The incorporation of linoleic
acid occurred to the highest degree in the choline phosphoglycerides.
The increases in the linoleic acid of the glycerophospholipids were
associated with decreased PF-3 activity. Studies of a similar nature in pigs by Andreoli and Miras (1) show even more extensive
modification of platelet fatty acids, reflecting the fatty acid
composition of the diet. In a report of studies on platelet lipids
in 3 population groups, namely, in Milan, Sicily, and Cincinnati
(10), it was found that platelet PS was relatively constant in the
3 regions and increased only slightly with age (Table I). Within
regions, however, stearic acid of PS was highest in the platelets
of Cincinnatians, lowest in the Sicilians, with the Milanese samples having intermediate levels. Although the stearic acid of PS
of the Sicilian samples was low, the palmitic acid content was relatively high (average 15%) and could have made up for the decreased stearic acid. Palmitic acid of PS of the Cincinnati subjects
was present in trace amounts; the Milanese samples had an intermediate level (average 4.4%). The polyunsaturated fatty acids of
PS of the 3 regions showed only slight variations. Based on rat
data (2), the platelet fatty acids of PS of the Cincinnati and Milanese populations could be interpreted as having a much higher
clotting activity than the Sicilian population.

In a study where a diet high in polyunsaturated fat (safflower
oil and margarine) was fed to healthy male subjects, the PS of platelets showed a decrease in stearate with a corresponding increase
in arachidonate in 3 of 4 subjects (11). When 3 male subjects were fed a diet high in saturated fat, stearic acid was increased in
platelet PS at the expense of the arachidonate. This lends further
support to the rat data of Gautheron and Renaud (2).

The role of dietary fat in predisposing thrombosis has been
given impetus by Hornstra. He demonstrated the induction of arterial thrombosis in rats and the use of the filtragometer technique
for evaluating the tendency to venous thrombosis in man. In rat
studies (6,7) where arterial thrombosis was evaluated by an arterial loop technique, it was found that the primary thrombogenic
components of the diet were myristic, palmitic, and stearic acids,
but that linoleic acid had an anti-thrombotic effect and oleic acid
a neutral effect. Fig. 3 shows the effect of sunflower-seed oil,
an oil rich in polyunsaturated fatty acids, on the thrombotic ob-

Table I. Fatty acid composition of phosphatidylserine of platelets[1]

Fatty Acids[4]	Area[2]			Age[3]		
	Milan	Cincinnati	Sicily	20-29	30-39	40-49
14:0	0.8±1.0	tr	0.6±0.5	0.3±0.6	0.7±1.1	0.4±0.4
16:0	4.4±1.0	0.2±0.4	15.0±4.9*	8.3±9.2	6.8±8.2	4.7±3.8
16:1	1.1±0.7	tr	1.4±0.4*	1.2±1.1	0.6±0.7	0.8±0.7
18:0	42.2±1.5	45.6±4.7	32.6±5.4*	37.7±7.4	42.5±10.6	41.4±6.6
18:1	25.8±2.9	34.9±1.3	26.1±5.1*	26.7±9.7	29.2±5.1	29.8±6.0
18:2	1.1±1.2	tr	2.7±1.0	1.5±2.0	0.8±1.6	1.4±1.2
20:0	1.1±1.1	tr	1.6±0.6	0.9±0.8	1.0±1.0	0.8±1.4
20:4	23.6±2.6	19.3±4.2	20.1±2.6	23.5±2.7	18.4±1.9	20.7±3.7

[1]Area percent of total fatty acids. [2]Mean ± SD for all composite samples in a given area. [3]Mean ± SD for all composite samples of the 3 areas for a given age group: the explanation for area and age data for all tables is similar. [4]14:0 (Myristic); 16:0 (Palmitic); 16:1 (Palmitoleic); 18:0 (Stearic); 18:1 (Oleic); 18:2 (Linoleic); 20:0 (Arachidic); 20:4 (Arachidonic).

*P<0.05.

(Courtesy of S. Karger, Basel, in "Dietary Fats and Thrombosis", 1974.)

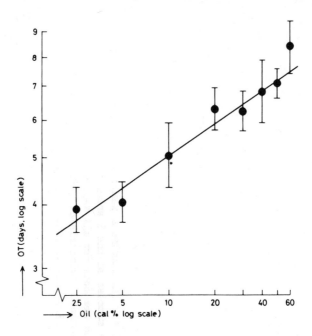

Fig. 3.   Influence of the dietary amount of sunflowerseed oil on thrombotic obstruction of the aorta-loop.   log OT = 0.481 + 0.2258 (log cal.% SO).   (Courtesy of G. Hornstra and A. Vendelmans-Starrenburg, Atherosclerosis 17, 369, 1973).

struction of the rat aorta loop.   The level of serum lipids seems to have no effect on the thrombotic tendency in rat and is in agreement with other findings that the cholesterol level of serum is unrelated to PF-3 activity, but that the ratio of saturated/polyunsaturated fatty acids is closely correlated with PF-3 activity (2).   Hornstra et al. (8) recently reported the influence of dietary fat on platelet function in man.   Through the use of a newly developed filter method, these authors demonstrated a decreased aggregability of platelets of men in a Finnish hospital where a high polyunsaturated fat diet (P/S ratio 1.6) was fed when compared with results in a hospital where a high saturated fat diet was fed (P/S ratio 0.25).

Using typical aggregating agents such as thrombin, collagen, and ADP, Renaud et al. (20) showed that the severity of thrombosis in rats fed high saturated fat diets was related to increased susceptibility to thrombin-induced aggregation but not to ADP- or collagen-induced aggregation.   In contrast, feeding a diet high in polyunsaturated fat did not show the thrombotic tendency or give increased thrombin aggregability of platelets in rats.

Of the various aggregating agesnts tested, increased thrombin-
induced aggregation was observed in 5 men who had definite signs of
coronary heart disease (20). Gondenfarb et al (3) found significantly increased platelet aggregation induced by ADP in men with a history of myocardial infarction. Steele et al (31) could find no instance of correlation of platelet aggregation with coronary artery
disease. In a dietary study in healthy men and women in the 40-60
age group (9), susceptibility to thrombin and collagen aggregation
was reduced markedly at the end of a 40-day feeding period of a diet
containing 25% fat calories and a P/S ratio of 1. Following a second 40-day feeding period on a diet containing 35% fat calories and
a P/S ratio of 1, the susceptibility to thrombin and collagen of the
same subjects returned to pre-dietary values. The results of the
aggregation tests suggest that the amount of fat in the diet is an
additional factor that must be taken into account in evaluating the
thrombogenic effect of dietary fats. How dietary fats influence
platelet aggregation is still obscure since the mechanisms involved
in aggregation tests have not been elucidated. It has been suggested (4) that alterations in the membrane fatty acids of platelets explain the aggregation changes, but considering the short term effects of diet on aggregation, it would seem very unlikely that membrane fatty acids would be altered to a great degree (11,18).

The fatty acid composition of platelet neutral lipids and phospholipids has been reported (14,18). Of the various phospholipids
present in platelets, all except the sphingomyelins are rich in linoleic and arachidonic acids. In a study of the platelet lipids of
3 populations, Cincinnati, Sicily, and Milan, it was found that the
beta-position of phosphatidylethanolamine (PE) had an unusually high
level of arachidonate, up to 95% in a single sample (Tables II and
III). One can speculate that the arachidonate of PE, along with its
structural role in biomembranes, may serve as a precursor of prostaglandins (PGs). PG biosynthesis in intact platelets has been demonstrated after stimulation with thrombin and collagen (28,29),
from ^{14}C-acetate (30), and by the conversion of ^{14}C-arachidonate
in lysed platelets (24). From these studies, it appears that human
platelets possess PG synthetase having properties similar to those
found in other tissues, especially in their in vitro requirement
for glutathione and hydroquinone (24).

Since PGE_2 has been well documented as being synthetized in a
number of tissues as well as in platelets, what is the source of
the essential fatty acids for their production? Considering the
known composition of phospholipids as rich sources of the essential
fatty acids, could they serve as precursors? It is known that the
production of PGs is limited by the availability of free arachidonate (12). The incorporation of linoleate and arachidonate into
platelet lipids was reported in human platelets (25), but it has
been reported that the level of free arachidonate is almost immeasur-
able (14). It appears that the platelet phospholipids could serve as
a reservoir for arachidonate. Assuming that this is the case, there

Table II.   Composition of total fatty acids of phosphatidylethanolamine of platelets[1]

Fatty[2] Acids	Area		
	Milan	Cincinnati	Sicily
16:0 DMA	5.2±2.7	5.3±2.3	6.5±2.0
16:0	5.0±1.9	8.0±3.2	6.7±1.2
16:1	1.7±1.2	2.2±2.7	1.4±0.7
18:0 DMA	9.9±6.4	6.2±4.2	7.2±2.4
18:0	21.7±3.7	18.2±3.6	23.8±7.0
18:1	10.9±2.9	9.0±1.0	12.0±1.2*
18:2	2.8±1.0	2.9±1.0	3.9±1.1
20:4	42.1±3.0	48.0±3.6	38.4±6.0

	Age		
	20–29	30–39	40–49
16:0 DMA	3.1±1.0	6.5±0.8	7.4±0.9**
16:0	8.8±2.3	5.9±2.3	5.0±0.5
16:1	3.5±1.5	0.7±0.6	1.2±0.3*
18:0 DMA	2.9±1.7	10.2±2.9	10.4±4.0*
18:0	23.8±9.0	20.3±1.1	19.4±1.3
18:1	12.6±2.1	9.9±1.5	9.5±1.5*
18:2	3.7±0.9	2.1±0.5	3.5±1.3*
20:4	40.8±10.5	44.3±2.1	43.4±2.2

[1]Area percent of total fatty acids.   [2]See Table I; 16:0 DMA (palmitaldehyde); 18:0 DMA (stearaldehyde).

*$P<0.05$; **$P<0.01$.

(Courtesy of S. Karger, Basel, in "Dietary Fats and Thrombosis", 1974.)

Table III. Composition of alpha- and beta-position fatty acids of phosphatidylethanolamine of platelets[1]

Area

Fatty[2] Acids	α-position			β-position		
	Milan	Cincinnati	Sicily	Milan	Cincinnati	Sicily
16:0 DMA	7.2±2.2	10.7±3.1	11.9±3.4	7.1±2.3	2.1±1.9	5.5±2.0
16:0	12.2±0.7	15.9±5.5	9.9±2.3	2.2±0.7	0.9±1.6	2.8±0.7
16:1	3.0±2.1	3.3±5.7	1.7±0.4			
18:0 DMA	11.3±5.2	11.9±6.7	13.0±5.8	9.0±4.4	1.1±1.0	6.3±5.0
18:0	39.4±8.8	43.3±7.4	42.9±7.4	11.2±3.0	6.9±2.2	13.0±2.9
18:1	14.4±1.1	13.2±2.4	11.6±1.5	6.8±4.5	4.1±1.0	5.5±1.2
18:2	1.4±1.2	tr	2.0±0.4	63.6±6.4	84.9±5.1	81.4±11.8
20:4	8.4±6.3	1.6±2.8	6.9±5.0			

Age

Fatty[2] Acids	α-position			β-position		
	20-29	30-39	40-49	20-29	30-39	40-49
16:0 DMA	6.2±1.4	13.0±1.8	14.8±4.8	6.3±3.0	4.7±4.3	3.8±0.6
16:0	11.3±6.9	7.1±1.4	6.2±1.4	4.1±1.7	1.4±1.2	2.1±0.4
16:1	2.9±4.2	1.0±1.0	0.5±1.6			
18:0 DMA	3.8±2.8	20.4±3.8	20.8±3.4	6.3±4.9	4.4±4.0	5.6±7.1
18:0	41.3±8.6	36.2±4.8	33.2±8.2	12.3±3.6	10.3±4.2	8.5±3.3
18:1	12.9±1.4	9.5±0.8	10.5±1.5	5.9±1.3	7.2±3.7	3.3±1.2
18:2	1.4±1.2	0.5±0.9	3.7±1.3	66.6±13.0	73.4±5.7	75.6±7.5
20:4	15.0±2.0	15.2±5.5	11.2±8.6			

[1]Area percent of total fatty acids. [2]See Table I; 16:0 DMA (palmitaldehyde); 18:0 DMA (Stearaldehyde).

(Courtesy of S. Karger, Basel, in "Dietary Fats and Thrombosis", 1974).

would be an obligatory requirement for phospholipase A_2. This enzyme has been demonstrated recently in platelets and has been shown to cleave 2-^{14}C-arachidonate from the parent labeled PE (26). The entire sequence of reactions leading to the biosynthesis of PGs from linoleate has been demonstrated, therefore, in human platelets.

The role of PGs in platelet metabolism is under investigation. PGE_2 may play a regulatory role in platelet metabolism by reducing cyclic AMP and PGE_1 stimulating the level of cyclic AMP. Since PGE_1 has an inhibitory effect on platelet aggregation and PGE_2 can either induce or inhibit platelet aggregation, depending on the level added to an in vitro medium, PGs may play important roles in thrombotic and inflammatory diseases (23). Very recently, when arachidonate was incubated in an in vitro platelet suspension it induced platelet aggregation. In the process, a contracting substance was generated that has been suggested to be a cyclic endoperoxide intermediate (34) formed during the biosynthesis of PGs but distinct from PGE_2 and PGF_2.

Another interesting characteristic of platelet PE is the presence of palmitaldehyde, stearaldehyde, and other plasmalogens (12). These alk-1-enyl type glycerophospholipids increased with age in the 3 population study (10) (Tables II and III). The functional significance of this type of fatty derivative is still unknown.

Changes in the pattern of phospholipids of platelets and red cells pose still another challenge to explain structural and metabolic characteristics of these blood components (10) (Table IV). When comparisons were made of the phospholipid patterns in the 3 population groups, differences related to geographical area were reported for both platelets and red cells. For example, the amount of PI of platelets of the Cincinnatians was considerably greater than that of the two other populations. Platelet PE, on the other hand, was highest in the Sicilian samples. The phospholipid pattern of the red cells related to region showed even greater differences. PE of red cells was lowest in the Cincinnatians compared to the other 2 groups; PS was highest in the Cincinnati samples. Explanations for the differences in the phospholipid pattern for platelets and red cells must await further experimentation. As the level of a single phospholipid changes, the contribution of its fatty acids to the composition of the total phospholipid is also altered. What are the functional or metabolic roles for these phospholipids apart from their structural characteristics? Are the differences in the lipids due to long-term nutritional adaptation or to genetic traits?

The observations on platelet phospholipids and phospholipid fatty acids in the studies reported above give clear indication that these changes were nutritionally induced. Even the changes that were related to age could be interpreted to have occurred as a consequence of long-term nutritional adaptation.

Table IV. Composition of platelets

	Area			Age		
	Milan	Cincinnati	Sicily	20-29	30-39	40-49
PRO (a)	58.1±1.4	58.1±1.8	57.3±5.2	59.7±0.6	58.4±2.4	55.4±3.5
TL (a)	19.2±4.7	19.5±1.9	19.4±0.9	20.9±3.6	18.7±1.9	18.4±2.6
CHOL (b)	24.2±2.8	24.2±2.7	20.4±3.0	20.7±3.1	22.7±3.3	25.0±1.8
PL (b)	65.3±6.2	62.2±4.2	63.5±7.3	59.7±3.3	63.1±3.7	68.3±3.2
PI (c)	6.8±0.5	11.2±1.6	6.0±0.8**	8.0±2.0	8.9±2.9	7.1±1.9
SPH	13.7±3.2	19.0±5.4	16.1±0.3	17.1±1.8	16.7±5.8	14.9±1.1
PC	28.7±1.0	29.3±4.8	32.4±1.3	31.4±1.7	28.0±3.6	31.0±1.6
PS	11.1±4.1	12.1±1.9	10.5±2.6	10.3±2.6	11.4±2.9	12.0±1.6
PE	18.0±2.3	16.7±0.9	23.5±0.8**	20.2±2.2	19.5±3.7	18.6±3.2
PA	3.9±2.0	6.0±0.4	2.3±1.0	4.3±2.1	3.5±1.6	4.4±1.8
CA	3.5±2.1	5.9±1.0	3.1±0.3	4.5±0.8	3.5±2.2	4.5±1.5

(a) % of total solids; (b) % of total lipids; (c) % of total lipid phosphorus.

**P<0.01.

PRO, Protein; TL, Total Lipid; CHOL, Cholesterol; PL, Phospholipid; PI,
Phosphatidylinositol; SPH, Sphingomyelin; PC, Phosphatidylcholine; PS,
Phosphatidylserine; PE, Phosphatidylethanolamine; PA, Phosphatidic Acid;
CA, Cardiolipin.

(Courtesy of S. Karger, Basel, in "Dietary Fats and Thrombosis", 1974.)

In conclusion, the nutritional changes reported suggest that high saturated fat diets predispose to thrombosis in experimental animals, and that this effect can be counteracted by feeding diets high in polyunsaturated fats. It appears that the high saturated fat diet influence the fatty acid composition of platelet phospholipids causing greater saturation and that the greater aggregability of the platelets is then mediated through PF-3.

REFERENCES

1. Andreoli, V.M. and Miras, C.J.
   Platelet lipids: Effects of a high fat or a high carbo-
   hydrate diet in pig plasma and platelet fatty acid composition.
   Life Sci. 10: 481, 1971.
2. Gautheron, P. and Renaud, S.
   Hyperlipemia induced hypercoagulable state in rat.
   Role of an increased activity of platelet phosphatidylserine
   response to certain dietary fatty acids.
   Thromb. Res. 1: 353, 1972.
3. Goldenfarb, P.B., Cathey M.H., Zucker, S.,
   Wilbur, P. and Corrigan, J.J.
   Changes in the hemostatic mechanism after myocardial
   infarction.
   Circulation 43: 538, 1971.
4. Gresham, G.A. and Howard, A.N.
   The independent production of atherosclerosis and
   thrombosis in rat.
   Brit. J. Exp. Path. 41: 395, 1960.
5. Hartroft, W.S. and O'Neal, R.N.
   Experimental production of coronary atherosclerosis.
   Amer. J. Cardiol. 9: 335, 1962.
6. Hornstra, G.
   The influence of dietary sunflowerseed oil and hardened
   coconut oil on intra-arterial occlusion thrombosis in rats.
   Nutr. Metabol. 13: 140, 1971.
7. Hornstra, G. and Vendelmans-Starrenburg, A.
   Induction of experimental arterial occlusive thrombi in rats.
   Atherosclerosis 17: 369, 1973.
8. Hornstra, G., Chait, A., Karnoven, M.J., Lewis, B.,
   Turpeinen, O. and Vergroesen, A.J.
   Influence of dietary fat on platelet function in men.
   Lancet 1: 1155, 1973.
9. Iacono, J.M., Binder, R.A., Jencks, J.A., Marshall, M.W.,
   Mackin, J.F., Canary, J.J., Waller, C. and Schoene, N.W.
   A test of the dietary recommendations of the Inter-society
   Commission for Heart Disease Resources: Platelet aggreg-
   ation and blood pressure.
   Circulat. Suppl. 4: 93, 1973.

10. Iacono, J.M., Zellner, D.C., Paoletti, R., Ishikawa, T.,
    Frigeni, V. and Fumagalli, R.
    A comparison of blood platelet and erythrocyte lipids
    in man in three age groups from three regions: Milan,
    Cincinnati, and Sicily.
    In: Dietary Fats and Thrombosis, ed. Renaud S. and Nordöy A.
    Basel, Karger, 1974.
11. Iacono, J.M. and Zellner, D.C.
    Unpublished observations.
12. Marcus, A.J., Ullman, H.L., Safier, L.B. and Ballard, H.S.
    Platelet phosphatides. Their fatty acid and aldehyde
    composition and activity in different clotting systems.
    J. Clin. Invest. 41: 2198, 1962.
13. Marcus, A.J.
    Platelet function: III.
    New Engl. J. Med. 280: 1330, 1969.
14. Marcus, A.J., Ullman, H.L. and Safier, L.B.
    Lipid composition of subcellular particles of human blood
    platelets.
    J. Lipid Res. 10: 108, 1969.
15. Mustard, J.F. and Murphy, E.A.
    Effect of different dietary fats on blood coagulation,
    platelet economy and blood lipids.
    Brit. Med. J. 1: 1651, 1962.
16. Mustard, J.F., Rowsell, H.C., Murphy, E.A. and Downie, H.G.
    Diet and thrombus formation.
    extracorporeal circulation in pigs.
    J. Clin. Invest. 42: 1783, 1963.
17. Nordöy, A. and Chandler, A.B.
    The influence of dietary fats on the adenosine diphosphate
    induced platelet thrombosis in the rat.
    Scand. J. Haemat. 1: 202, 1964.
18. Nordöy, A. and Rödset, J.M.
    The influence of dietary fats on platelets in man.
    Acta. Med. Scand. 190: 27, 1971.
19. Renaud, S. and Allard, D.
    Thrombosis in connection with serum lipid changes in the rat.
    Circulat. Res. 11: 388, 1962.
20. Renaud, S., Kuba, K., Goulet, C., Lemire, Y. and Allard, C.
    Relationship between platelet fatty acid composition and
    platelet aggregation in rat and man, in connection with
    thrombosis.
    Circulat. Res. 26: 553, 1970.
21. Renaud, S. and Lecompte, F.
    Hypercoagulability induced by hyperlipemia in rat, rabbit,
    and man.
    Role of Platelet Factor 3.

22. Renaud, S. and Gautheron, P.
    Dietary fats and experimental (cardiac and venous) thrombosis.
    In: Dietary Fats and Thrombosis, ed. Renaud S. and Nordöy A.
    Basel, Karger, 1974.
23. Salzman, E.W.
    Cyclic AMP and platelet function.
    New Engl. J. Med. 286: 358, 1972.
24. Schoene, N.W. and Iacono, J.M.
    Use of lysed human platelets to study PGE$_2$ production.
    Prostaglandins.
    In press.
25. Schoene, N.W. and Iacono, J.M.
    Metabolism of linoleic and arachidonic acids in
    human blood platelets.
    Fed. Proc. 32: 919, 1973.
26. Schoene, N.W. and Iacono, J.M.
    Phospholipase A$_2$ activity in lysed human platelets.
    Fed. Proc.
    In press.
27. Slotta, K.H.
    Thromboplastin. I. Phospholipid moiety of thromboplastin.
    Proc. Soc. Exp. Biol. Med. 103: 53, 1960.
28. Smith, J.B. and Willis, A.L.
    Formation and release of prostaglandins by platelets
    in response to thrombin.
    Brit. J. Pharmacol. 40: 545, 1970.
29. Smith, J.B., Ingerman, C., Kocsis, J.J. and Silver, M.J.
    Formation of prostaglandins during aggregation of human
    blood platelets.
    J. Clin. Invest. 52: 965, 1973.
30. Srivastava, K.C. and Clausen, J.
    Synthesis of prostaglandins (PGE, PGF, PGA, PGB)
    in human platelets.
    Lipids 7: 762, 1972.
31. Steele, P.P., Weily, H.S., Davies, H. and Genton, E.
    Platelet function studies in coronary artery disease.
    Circulation 48: 1194, 1973.
32. Therriault D., Nichols, T. and Jensen, H.
    Purification and identification of brain phospholipids
    associated with thromboplastic activity.
    J. Biol. Chem. 233: 1061, 1958.
33. Thomas, W.A. and Hartroft, W.S.
    Myocardial infarction in rats fed high fat and cholesterol
    diets containing thiouracil and sodium cholate.
    Circulation 19: 65, 1959.
34. Vargaftig, B.B. and Zirnis, P.
    Platelet aggregation induced by arachidonic acid is
    accompanied by release of potential inflammatory mediators
    distinct from PGE$_2$ and PGF$_2$.
    Nature New Biol. 244: 114, 1973.

PREVENTION OF ATHEROSCLEROSIS BY DIET

PRESENT STATE AND CONCLUSIONS

J.C. SOMOGYI

Institute for Nutrition Research, Rüschlikon-Zürich

The connection between atherosclerosis and certain nutrients was discussed extremely well in several lectures of this seminar. In the following an attempt will be made to summarize the present state of this topic and draw some conclusions, as to how athero-sclerosis can be prevented by dietary means.

Dealing with this matter I think it best if we go through the various nutrients individually and discuss their role in the pre-vention and, if necessary, in the pathogenesis of atherosclerosis. Some of them only briefly, others from this point of view, the more important ones, in greater detail.

According to our present knowledge proteins are not involved in the genesis of cardiovascular diseases of atherosclerotic origin. Quite to the contrary some of our protein sources such as lean meat, lean fish, skim milk, etc. are widely used in diets for the preven-tion of coronary heart disease as well as in connection with the therapy of these diseases.

It is interesting to mention that in animal experiments several investigators found that the serum cholesterol content was decreas-ed by a well balanced amino acid supply. According to Mann et al. (1960) (1), deficiency of sulfur-containing amino acids connected with a cholesterol rich diet caused hypercholesterolemia in monkeys. These results could not be confirmed by others. In any case amino acids do not seem to play an important role in atherosclerotic pro-cesses.

Yudkin (1964) (2) (1968) (3), Macdonald (1971) (4) (1972) (5), Albrink (1973) (6), Kritchevsky (1973) (7) and Heinle et al. (1969) (8) dealt among others with the question whether carbohydrates, especially sucrose and fructose, are of major importance in the origin of atherosclerosis. We have heard the excellent lecture of Dr. Kritchevski and Prof. MacDonald so I do not need to go into this topic in detail.

But it seems to be that 1) only certain carbohydrates may play a role in atherosclerosis and 2) only in a certain group of the population, which is "carbohydrate sensitive" i.e. up to 13% of men between 25-79 years respond with an elevation of blood triglycerides and in some group of women, 3) over-abundance of carbohydrates in the diet may be the prerequisite. 4) carbohydrates may have an effect only after they are transformed to triglycerides in the organism.

It is interesting to mention that according to Paul et al. (1968) (9) the statistical analysis of their investigation with a coronary and non-coronary group has shown no significant association between heavy intake of sucrose and coronary disease.

Since on the other hand overweight is indirectly one of the risk factors of atherosclerosis, especially of heart infarction, it is of advantage to recommend a moderate intake of carbohydrates for the dietary prevention of coronary heart disease. This should be taken into consideration even if it would lack the final proof e.g. by epidemiological investigations for the importance of certain sugars in the pathogenesis of atherosclerotic disease.

At this point may I say a few words about the risk factors which play a role in atherosclerosis. As it is known the major risk factors are the following: high serum cholesterol level or more generally expressed hyperlipidemia, hypertension and cigarette smoking. Fig. 1 shows the relation between morbidity of coronary heart disease and these risk factors (33).

As you can see, in persons with one risk factor heart infarction and sudden death doubles, with two risk factors triples and in those with three risk factors these events are ten times more frequent, than in individuals who do not smoke and have "normal" (physiological) cholesterol and blood pressure values.

Furthermore there are other risk factors - some viewing them of minor significance - including: heredity, stress, hormonal disturbances, obesity and insufficient physical activity. It seems to others and also to me that the latter two are rather important in the genesis of coronary disease.

According to the recently published Stockholm prospective study by Carlson and Böttiger (1972 (10) plasma cholesterol and plasma triglycerides "are risk factors for ischaemic heart disease independent of each other, and a combined elevation of these two plasma lipids carries the highest risk for ischaemic heart disease".

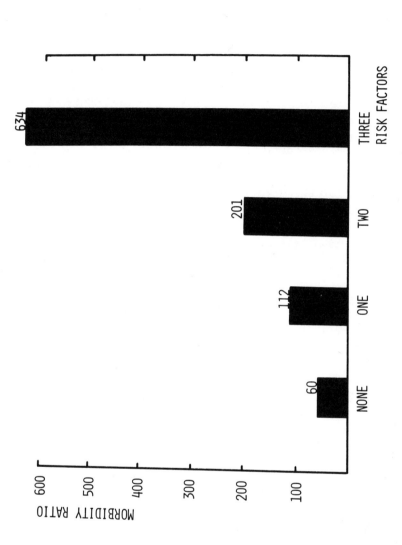

Fig. 1. The relationship between coronary heart disease and the risk factors: high serum cholesterol, hypertension and excessive cigarette smoking.

Also the early retrospective studies of Albrink (1961) (11) suggested that hypertriglyceridemia is a significant risk factor in atherosclerotic heart disease.

Let us now follow with the role of the dietary fats in these occurrences.

There is convincing evidence for the great importance of the quality and to some extent also the quantity of dietary fats in the pathogenesis and prevention of atherosclerosis. Discussing the question of how atherosclerosis, and especially coronary heart disease, is influenced by dietary means, there are two groups of substances of specific interest: cholesterol and polyunsaturated fatty acids.

In connection with cholesterol I would like to deal briefly with the role of dietary cholesterol. Our point of view in this matter has been changed repeatedly in the course of the last few years. About 15-20 years ago it was generally accepted that the cholesterol content of the diet is a major factor for the serum cholesterol level in man.

But after it was established that exogenous cholesterol makes up only a small portion of that which is synthesized by the organism, it was believed that dietary cholesterol could be neglected, with the exception of extremely high intakes. This idea was strengthened when it was thought that also in man cholesterol synthesis is inhibited by dietary cholesterol by a feed-back mechanism, as described in dogs (Gould and Taylor (1950)) (12) and rats (Tomkins et al. (1953)) (13). We know now that even high dosages of cholesterol, e.g. 2 g, do not decrease cholesterol synthesis in the human liver.

The investigations which were carried out between 1960-68 a.o. by Beveridge et al. (14,15), Wells and Bronte-Stewart (16), Keys and co-workers (17), Hodges and co-workers (18) Hedgsted et al. (19) have shown however, that dietary cholesterol intake, if it exceeds a certain level, can also cause an increase in serum cholesterol.

The concept still remains valid that the serum cholesterol level depends primarily on the composition of the fats, more exactly on the ratio of polyunsaturated to saturated fatty acids in the food. But according to several authors and to the recommendations of the American Heart Association and other medical organizations, cholesterol intake should be reduced to 300 mg/day in persons with high serum cholesterol levels. Such a dietetic measure seems to be rather important in countries in which the dietary cholesterol intake, due to the eating havits, is generally high, e.g. in the U.S.A., where about 650 mg cholesterol is consumed per day per capita (Dayton et al. (1969)) (36); in other countries e.g. in Switzerland the daily intake is much lower e.g., between about 300-400 mg/day/capita.

It can be calculated by the formula described by Keys and co-workers (1965) (20) and Thomasson et al. (1967) (21), that 100 mg dietary cholesterol cause an increase of about 6 mg % of serum cholesterol.

This means, that for example a regular daily intake of 1 egg containing about 300 mg cholesterol, raises the serum cholesterol by 18 mg %, i.e. nearly 10% of the so called "normal" serum cholesterol value.

It is however not difficult to reduce dietary cholesterol since there are only few food items with rather a high content of cholesterol which have to be omitted (Table I).

Egg yolk, brain, viscera and certain crustacea contain high concentrations of cholesterol, as can be taken from Table I.

In this connection may I mention that according to Adlersberg et al. (1956) (23) serum cholesterol level rises with increasing age, and a sex dependent difference has also been observed (Fig. 2).

The serum cholesterol of man rises at the age of 25-27 and tends to remain at this level for the following years. This is in contrast to female subjects where the serum cholesterol shows a continuous increase, reaching a maximum at about 57 years.

A few years ago, we carried out similar investigations with 200 women Somogyi (1964) (24), (1969) (25). The results of a group of 80 female subjects are summarized in Fig. 3.

The participants were recruited from middle-aged and elderly residents and nurses of a convalescent home. Persons with a history of diabetes or acute diseases were excluded from this study. The other part of this investigation vas carried out with 120 healthy females in a mental home.

All participants received the same diet in which the content of fats, proteins and polyunsaturated fatty acids was determined, the carbohydrate content was obtained from food tables and the caloric value was calculated. Age groups were formed with 8-10 subjects. The youngest group had an average age of 22 years, the eldest of 88 years. Each point of this curve represents the mean of the serum cholesterol values of subjects of each age group.

There are several possibilities for explaining the decrease of the serum cholesterol levels in the groups over sixty years. One reason could be that the mortality of subjects with a high serum cholesterol content is greater, they die earlier and therefore the mean of each group over sixty is gradually reduced.

May I now deal briefly with the role of the polyunsaturated fatty acids in the prevention of coronary heart disease and with the cardinal question whether the importance of the dietary fats as causative and/or preventive factor of atherosclerosis is proved, or whether other nutrients are more responsible for this disease.

Table I.   Cholesterol content of various foods

Food	mg/100 g edible portion	Remarks
Eggs		
whole	470	
yolk	1,800	
white	0	
Organs/various		
Brain	2,200	
Heart	150	
Liver	300	
Thymus	300	
Meat		
Beef	125^	^without bones
Veal	90^	
Pork	70^	
Chicken	60^	
Lamb	70^	
Fish various	70	
Milk products		
Curd (cottage cheese)	15	
Butter	250	
Cheese:		
Camembert	140	
Emmental	145	
Limburg	135	
Parmesan	190	
Tilsit	140	
Shell fish		
Lobster	200^	^meat only
Shrimps	125^	
Oysters	200^	
Mussels	150^	
Caviar	300	

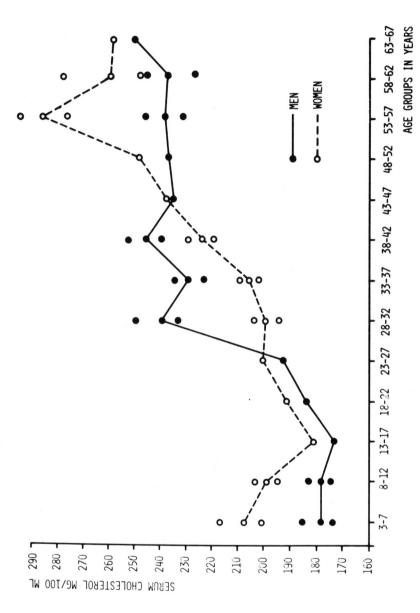

Fig. 2. Changes of the serum cholesterol level of men and women with increasing age.

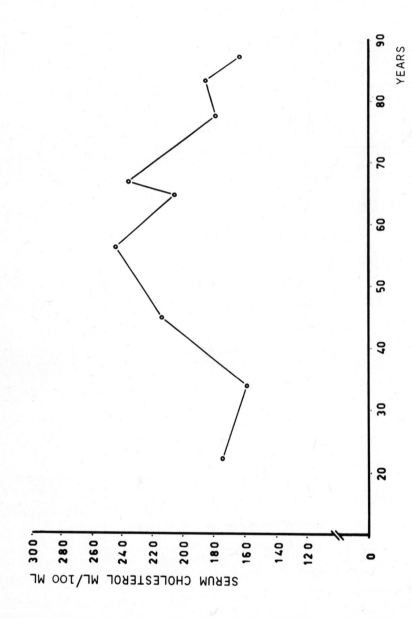

The primary importance of the polyunsaturated fatty acids in the regulation, more exactly in lowering the serum cholesterol level in man was demonstrated a.o. by the early experiments of Bronte-Stewart et al. (1956) (26). According to these investigations the increase of the cholesterol level caused by saturated fatty acids or by eggs can be diminished by simultaneous intake of sunflower oil or olive oil (Fig. 4).

These experiments have also shown that not the total fat consumptio - the fat intake was doubled by the additional supply of sunflower oil - but the composition of the dietary fats i.e. the ratio of polyunsaturated fatty acids to saturated fats plays the more important role in these interrelations.

If the fat consumption and therefore the content of saturated fatty acids in the diet is low, the serum cholesterol can remain at a moderate level, as was observed in the peoples of the Near East e.g. the Yemenites, who consume almost exclusively saturated fats, but their total fat consumption is very low. This observation is not in disagreement with the concept which I mentioned before.

The early epidemiological investigations of F.A.O. (1955) (27) and W.H.O. (1956) (28), the international cross sectional epidemiological studies of Keys (1956) (29) (1970) (30), as well as a great number of recent investigations proved the decrease of serum cholesterol by essential fatty acids to be connected with a marked decline of morbidity and mortality by coronary heart disease.

I would like to list in this connection the following investigations: the interesting prospective Framingham Study by Kagan, Dawber et al. (1962) (31), the Anti-Coronary-Club Study of Joliffe et al. (1963) (32) and Christakis et al. (1966) (33), and that of Leren (1966) (34) in Norway, the National-Diet-Heart Study in the U.S.A. (1968) (35), the clinical trials of Dayton et al. (1969) (36) and the important clinical-epidemiological investigations of Turpeinen, Karvonen and Roine (1967) (37) which have been recently finalized after 12 years (by Miettinen, Turpeinen et al. (1972) (38). In this connection is to be mentioned that Fidanza (1972) (73) summarized in a recent paper the epidemiological investigations on the relation between dietary fats and atherosclerosis.

It would be interesting to deal with these important investigations in more detail, but this is outside of the scope of such a paper. I would like to summarize only the results of investigations of Turpeinen et al. (1972) (38). This study, in agreement with many others and shows impressively that a reduction of serum cholesterol level by dietary means is connected with a marked decrease in the incidence of coronary heart disease.

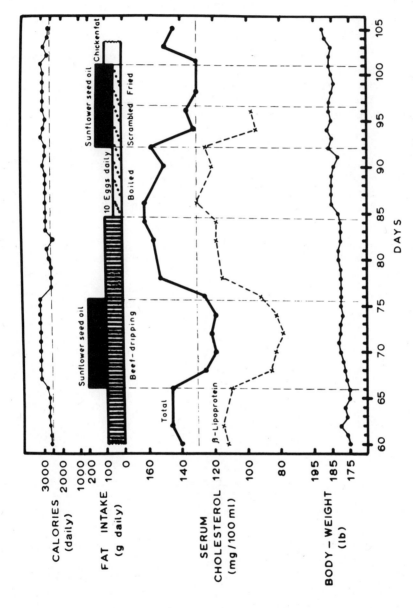

Fig. 4.   The effect of simultaneous intake of sunflower oil and saturated
fats on the serum cholesterol level.

The study was done in two mental hospitals. A cross over design was used. From 1959 to 1965 hospital N had a cholesterol-lowering diet, whereas hospital K had the usual Finnish diet. In 1965 the diets were reversed. The residents of hospital K received a cholesterol-lowering diet (P/S ratio 1.42-1.78) and those of hospital N the normal Finnish diet (P/S ratio 0.26). The second period lasted from 1965 to 1971. The results of this investigation are summarized in Fig. 5, Table II and Table III.

In the experimental group (hospital N) a significant drop of serum cholesterol was observed after a few months; this value remained constant for the following six years. After changing the diet in 1965 the serum cholesterol rose within an year and remained on this level until 1971, i.e. the end of the second period. An opposite behaviour was observed in the men in hospital K (Fig. 5 and Table II).

In men the use of cholesterol lowering diet was associated with a significantly reduced incidence of coronary heart disease (Table III).

This investigation, among others, supports to close connection between nutrition, serum cholesterol level and coronary heart disease.

The requirement of polyunsaturated fatty acids is high. It is estimated that 4-7 g per day is needed. According to a recent publication by Wolfram and Zöllner (1971) (39) it is even more: namely 9.3 g per day at a daily calorie intake of 2600. According to Holman (1962) (40), the minimum linoleate requirement should amount to 2% of total calories.

The fulfilment of the requirement of polyenic acids is generally easy, if the diet is prepared with oils containing a high portion of polyunsaturated fatty acids, e.g. sunflower, soyabean oil, corn oil, safflower oil, wheat germ oil etc. The situation becomes more difficult if a greater intake is needed because an elevated serum cholesterol level has to be reduced. According to Zöllner's recent unpublished investigation (1973) (41) 70 g sunflower or olive oil per day is necessary for this purpose. This may cause some complication in the diet due to its high calorie content. In my experience this can also be achieved with a smaller intake of about 40 g/day.

It is striking that olive oil, with only 8-10% polyenic acids, has the same effect as sunflower oil with 50-60% PUFA. It seems that in olive oil an unknown factor or factors are contained which decrease the cholesterol content of blood.

May I deal with two practical questions which are connected with this problem and are often asked by patients. 1) Are the extracted refined oils and the so called cold pressed oils equivalent in respect of their content of polyunsaturated fatty acids?

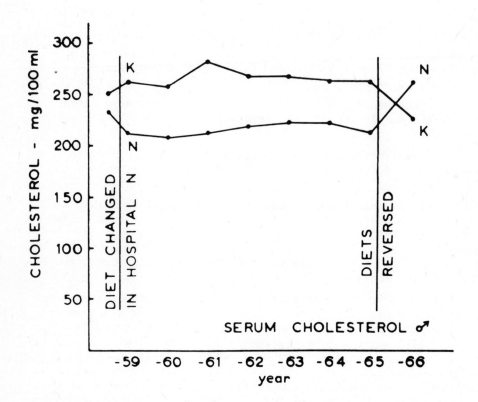

Fig. 5.   Mean cholesterol levels of men in two hospitals.

Table II. Mean serum cholesterol values

HOSPITAL	SERUM CHOLESTEROL MG/100 ML		
	1ST PERIOD	2ND PERIOD	DIFFERENCE
MALES			
N	217	266	49
K	268	234	34
FEMALES			
N	245	278	33
K	270	236	34

Table III. Incidence of coronary heart disease

PATIENTS	HOSPITAL	
	N	K
AT RISK	313	241
DEVELOPED CORONARY HEART DISEASE^	17	30
ANNUAL INCIDENCE PER 1000	14.4	33.0

^ Criteria: Electrocardiographic evidence or "coronary" death.

2) The second question is whether the essential fatty acids are destroyed by heating, for instance, by frying or roasting?

A few years ago we carried out experiments in this direction with sunflower oil in my institute.

We determined the polyenic acid and the vitamin E content in seven brands of cold pressed sunflower oil and in four brands of extracted, refined sunflower oil (Table IV).

As is shown by Table IV there is no significant difference in the concentration of polyunsaturated fatty acids and vitamin E between the two types of oils.

Also the heating of sunflower oil for two hours at a temperature of 210°C did not cause a decrease in the linoleic and linolenic acid content (Fig. 6).

These results are of some practical importance because they show that sunflower and similar oils can also be used for frying and roasting. This helps to cover the requirement of polyunsaturated fatty acids.

Vitamins are generally not important in the prevention of atherosclerosis, as can be concluded among others from the investigations of Schettler and his colleagues (1960) (42). They were carried out in seven clinics in Germany and the effect of high doses of vitamin A, vitamin E and pyridoxine (A: 60-120,000 I.U./day E: 140-200 mg/day, B₆: 60-120 mg/day) was tested during a year in patients with atherosclerotic cardiovascular diseases. No objective improvement was observed.

It is to point out that all the vitamins proposed for the treatment of coronary heart disease or of single symptoms e.g. for decrease of the elevated serum cholesterol level, were used in much higher doses (1:10-1:400), than the daily requirement. The effect is, if any, pharmacological, and not dietary.

An exception is vitamin E, but not for the reasons proposed by W.E. Shute (1972) (43) in his best-seller book. High intake of polyenic acids can cause a vitamin E deficiency in experimental animals and man, mainly if the vitamin E content of food is marginal.

Wiss and co-workers (1964) (44) as well as Weber and Weiser (1967) (45) clarified the relationship between vitamin E requirement and intake of linoleic acid by the hemolysis test. According to these authors man needs 0.5 to 1.0 mg vitamin E per gram linoleic acid to compensate for the increased requirement of vitamin E due to higher polyenic acid content in such diets. Only therefore and not "for ailing and healthy hearts" can a daily intake of 10-15 mg vitamin E be recommended.

Table IV. Polyunsaturated fatty acid and vitamin E content in
cold pressed and extracted, refined sunflower oils

	PUFA in %	Vitamin E in mg %
Cold pressed:		
Brand 1	65.3	70.7
Brand 2		70.5
Brand 3	64.5	75.5
Brand 4	61.4	76.6
Brand 5	59.4	
Brand 6	61.7	58.0
Brand 7	62.8	68.4
Mean:	62.5	69.9
Extr. refin.:		
Brand 1	61.2	66.1
Brand 2	59.3	64.5
Brand 3	57.8	69.0
Brand 4	59.4	62.1
Mean:	59.4	65.4

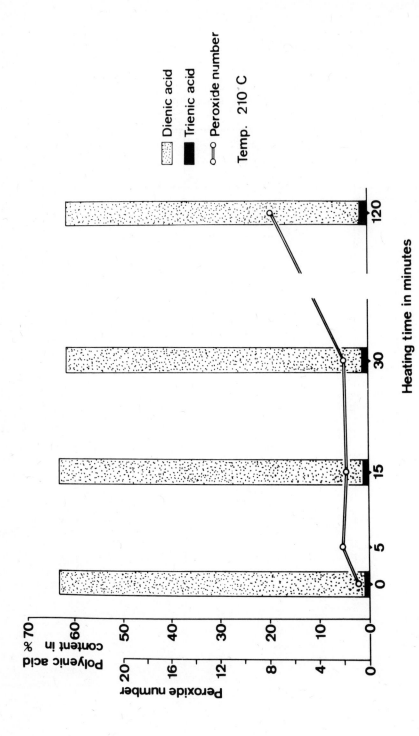

Fig. 6.   The influence of heating on the polyenic acid content of sunflower oil.

Table V. Daily requirement and recommended dosage of various
vitamins for the decrease of serum cholesterol levels

Vitamin	Daily requirement	Dosage	Ratio Requirem.: Dose	Decrease of serum cholesterol
Niacin	15 mg	3-6 g	1:200-1:400	+
B_6	1-2 mg	25 mg	1:12 -1:25	-
		60 mg	1:30 -1:60	-
A	5000 IE	60000 IE	1:12	±
E	10-15 mg	140 mg	1:9 -1:14	-

Table VI. Mean percentage changes in death rate between 1948-
1954 and 1958-1964 as function of change in water hardness^

Cause of death	Water hardness		
	increase[1]	no change[2]	decrease[3]
cardiovascular	8,5%	11,2%	20,2%
other causes	- 10,8%	- 13,0%	- 12,4%

^ Male population 45-64 years of age in England and Wales
   1 = 5 towns   2 = 72 towns   3 = 6 towns.

   Crawford, M.D. et al., Lancet 2: 327, 1971.

Some minerals and trace elements either inhibit or enhance the development of cardiovascular diseases. Available data suggest that death rates for cardiovascular disease of atherosclerotic origin are inversely related to hardness of drinking water, as is shown also by Table VI.

In many countries it has been found that the harder the drinkking water, the lower the mortality of cardiovascular disease, so Schroeder (1960) (46) in the U.S.A., Morris and co-worker (1961) (47) in England and Wales, Björck et al. (1965) (48) in Sweden, Masironi (1970) (49) etc. It is interesting to mention that Kobayashi (50) from Japan was probably the first in 1957 to suggest that water might be related to death rates from cardiovascular disease.

The close relationship of this disease to water quality could be explained by several mechanisms for instance hard water could be protective, because its calcium - magnesium - and/or trace elements content or soft water could contain toxic elements e.g. metal contaminants from distribution pipes. Very little is known about the latter.

More data is available on the effect of the above mentioned minerals. It is suggested that the protective effect of hard water is mainly due to its calcium and magnesium content.

According to Masironi et al. (1972) (51) calcium could be important in two ways. "First it might inhibit" - I cite now Masironi - "the absorption of harmful elements from pipes and soil, or calcium ions might be an addition to dietary calcium". This latter concept is supported by the observation that low serum calcium concentrations were found in soft water areas (Bierenbaum et al. (1969) (52), Kamiyama et al. (1969) (53).

A low intake of magnesium may also contribute to a higher mortality of cardiovascular disease in soft water areas. Magnesium - and also calcium - are involved in enzyme systems in the heart muscle. Sealig (1972) (54) has shown for example that inadequate magnesium concentration interferes with the activation of adenosintriphosphatase and causes a loss of potassium by myocardial cells. This might be responsible for sudden death from coronary artery disease.

According to Crawford (1973) (55,56) a balanced intake of the ratio $\frac{Ca + Mg}{Na}$ may be important to the stability of electrolyte balance.

"A decrease in this ratio may contribute both to the prevalence of hypertension and to the increased risk of sudden death in people with coronary heart disease".

From the trace elements, cadmium seems to be a factor in human hypertension (Schroeder and Vinton (1962) (57), Schroeder (1965) (58).

Cadmium became suspect as a cause of hypertension because of its specific affinity to the kidneys, which - as it is known - plays an important role in the control of blood pressure. According to Schroeder (1965) (58) the cadmium content of kidneys of hypertensive subjects is significantly higher than that of similar normotensive persons: 4,220 g cadmium/ 1 g kidney ash against 2940 g. The difference is highly significant (p=0.0005).

In contrast to that chromium seems to be efficient against atherosclerosis. Sugar causes mobilisation of chromium in the body connected with significant losses in the urine.

The typical diet in North America and in Europe lacks chromium. This is due to the very low content of chromium in refined food (sugar, flour) consumed in excess in the industrialized countries (Schroeder (1967)) (59). The chromium level in human tissues, including aorta, decreases with age (Schroeder (1968)) (60). Foods with a higher content of chromium e.g. whole wheat bread, might be recommended to persons with cardiovascular disease, although no definite proof exists for this interrelation.

Interesting is the contradiction concerning the effect of copper in atherosclerosis. While in previous investigations by Kanabrocki and co-workers (1965) (61), (1967) (62) a slight increase of serum copper and significant increase in the urine of patients with heart infarction was observed and according to Harman (1966) (63), (1968) (64) copper enhances the experimental atherosclerosis. In a recent publication of Coulson (1973) (65) an inverse effect of copper is described. In young pigs with copper deficiency after about 100 days of life serious lesions in the heart and great vessels were formed. These include a.o. occlusive dissecting aneurisms of the coronary arteries, myocardial infarction, rupture of the aorta, etc. The aorta of the most seriously affected animals may contain lesions throughout their length.

It seems to be that vanadium reduces the cholesterol level in plasma and in the aorta in rabbits as well as in healthy persons (Mountain et al. (1956 (66), Schütte (1964) (67), Korkhov (1965) (68). This effect is due to an inhibition of the cholesterol synthesis (Schroeder et al. (1963) (69), Speckmann and Brink (1967) (70) at the level of mevalonic acid (Curran et al. (1959) (71). Schroeder (1966) (72) found "a significant negative correlation between the vanadium content" of drinking water and mortality of coronary heart disease.

In conclusion it is to emphasize that atherosclerosis can be regarded as a disease of multiple etiology. I mentioned at the beginning of this paper the various predisposing factors. There is no doubt that for prevention diet and physical activity play an important role.

In spite of some differences concerning the importance of different nutrients in its pathogenesis, the recommendations of various medical and nutritional organizations and research workers for the prevention of coronary heart disease by dietary means show a good agreement.

They recommend:

1) reduction of calories in case of overweight;
2) reduction of fat consumption from 40% to 25-30% of the total calorie intake;
3) reduction of the content of saturated fatty acids and an increase of polyunsaturated fatty acids in the diet;
4) limitation of the cholesterol content in the food which "for all practical purposes means less egg yolk" - as Stare (1964) (22) expressed it a bit sharply;
5) moderate supply of carbohydrates;
6) increase of consumption of not refined foods, of fruits, vegetables, potatoes, lean meat and lean fish according to the Swedish Medical and Nutrition Societies;
7) a reduction of sodium chloride intake to 5 g/day is also of advantage.

I have made the attempt to point out the solved and unsolved problems about the relationship between nutrition and atherosclerosis. If this paper gives impulses to discussions and further research in this field, then its objectives have been reached.

REFERENCES

1. Mann, G.V., McNally, A. and Prudhomme, C.:
   Experimental atherosclerosis. Effects of sulfur compounds on hypercholesteremia and growth in cysteine deficient monkeys.
   Amer. J. Clin. Nutr. 8: 491, 1960.
2. Yudkin, J.:
   Dietary fat and dietary sugar in relation to ischaemic heart-disease and diabetes.
   Lancet 2: 4, 1964.
3. Yudkin, J.:
   Dietary and serum-cholesterol.
   Lancet 1: 917, 1968).
4. MacDonald, I.:
   Dietary carbohydrates and blood lipids.
   Nutrition and cardiovascular diseases. Proc. VII Int. Meeting of the Centro Studi Lipidi, Rimini 1970, p. 80.
   (Morgagni Edizioni Scientifiche, Roma 1971).

5. Macdonald, I;:
   Atheroma in various forms of essential hyperlipidaemia.
   Sugar and human health.
   4th Int. Sugar Research Symp. Zurich, 1972.
6. Albrink, M.J.:
   Triglyceridemia.
   J. Amer. Diet. Ass. 62: 626, 1973.
7. Kritchevsky, D.:
   The effects of feeding various carbohydrates
   on the development of hypercholesterolemia and
   atherosclerosis.
   Proc. Int. Meeting on Diet and atherosclerosis,Rome, 1973
   In press.
8. Heinle, R.A., Levy, R.I., Fredrickson, D.S. and Gorlin, R.:
   Lipid and carbohydrate abnormalities in patients with
   angiographically documented coronary artery disease.
   Amer. J. Cardiol. 24: 178, 1969.
9. Paul, O., McMillan, A., McKean, H. and Park, H.:
   Sucrose intake and coronary heart-disease.
   Lancet, 2: 1049, 1968.
10. Carlson, L.A. and Böttiger, L.E.:
    Ischaemic heart-disease in relation to fasting values of
    plasma triglycerides and cholesterol.
    Stockholm Prospective Study.
    Lancet, 1: 865, 1972.
11. Albrink, M.J., Meigs, J.W. and Man, E.B.:
    Serum lipids, hypertension and coronary artery disease.
    Amer. J. Med. 31: 4, 1961.
12. Gould, R.G. and Taylor, C.B.:
    Effect of dietary cholesterol on hepatic cholesterol synthesis.
    Fed. Proc. 9: 179, 1950.
13. Tomkins, G.M., Sheppard, H. and Chaikoff, I.L.:
    Cholesterol synthesis by liver. III. Its regulation
    by ingested cholesterol.
    J. Biol. Chem. 201: 137, 1953.
14. Beveridge, J.M.R., Connell, W.F., Haust, H.L. and Mayer, G.A.:
    Dietary cholesterol and plasma cholesterol levels in man.
    Canad. J. Biochem. Physiol. 37: 575, 1959.
15. Beveridge, J.M.R., Connell, W.F., Mayer, G.A. and Haust, H.L.:
    The response of man to dietary cholesterol.
    J. Nutr. 71: 61, 1960.
16. Wells, V.M. and Bronte-Stewart, B.:
    Egg yolk and serum cholesterol levels:
    Importance of dietary cholesterol intake.
    Brit. Med. J . 1: 577, 1963.
17. Keys, A., Anderson, J.T. and Grande, F.:
    Serum cholesterol response to changes in the diet.
    II. The effect of cholesterol in the diet.
    Metabolism, 14: 759, 1965.

18. Connor, W.E., Stone, D.B. and Hodges, R.E.:
    The interrelated effects of dietary cholesterol and
    fat upon human serum lipid levels.
    J. Clin. Invest. 43: 1691, 1964.
19. Hegsted, D.M., McGandy, R.B., Myers, M.L. and Stare, F.J.:
    Quantitative effects of dietary fat on serum cholesterol
    in man.
    Amer. J. Clin. Nutr. 17: 281, 1965.
20. Grande, F., Anderson, J.T., Chlouverakis, C.,
    Proja, M. and Keys, A.:
    Effect of dietary cholesterol on man's serum lipids.
    J. Nutr. 87: 52, 1965.
21. Thomasson, H.J., De Boer, J. and De Iongh, H.:
    Influence of dietary fats on plasma lipids.
    Path. Microbiol. 30: 629, 1967.
22. Stare, F.J.:
    Nutritional suggestions for the primary prevention
    of coronary heart disease.
    J. Amer. Diet. Ass. 48: 88, 1966.
23. Adlersberg, D., Schaefer, L.E., Steinberg, A.G. and
    Chung-I-Wang:
    Age, Sex, Serum-lipids and coronary atherosclerosis.
    J. Amer. Med. Ass.: 192: 619, 1956.
24. Somogyi, J.C.:
    Unpublished experiments (1964).
25. Somogyi, J.C.:
    Ernährung und Atherosklerose
    Bibl. "Nutr.Diet." 12: 11, 1969.
26. Bronte-Stewart, B., Antonis, A., Eales, L. and Brock, J.F.:
    Effects of feeding different fats on serum-cholesterol level.
    Lancet, 1: 521, 1956.
27. Food and Agriculture Organization of the United Nations:
    Food Balance Sheets. FAO, Rome, 1955.
28. World Health Organization:
    Epidem. Vital. Statist. Rep. 9: 358, 1956.
29. Keys, A.:
    The diet and the development of coronary heart disease.
    J. Chron. Dis. 4: 364, 1956.
30. Keys, A.:
    Prospects for the control of coronary heart disease as
    deduced from comparison of populations.
    Proc. VII Int. Meeting of the Centro Studi Lipidi, Rimini, 1970,
    p. 175 - Morgagni Edizioni Scientifiche, Roma, 1971.
31. Jolliffe, N., Baumgartner, L., Rinzler, S.H., Archer, M.,
    Stephenson, J.H. and Christakis, G.J.:
    The Anti-Coronary Club: The first four years.
    N.Y. St. J. Med. 63: 1, 1963.

32. Christakis, G., Rinzler, S.H., Archer, M., Winslow, G.,
    Jampel, S., Stephenson, J., Friedman, G., Fein, H.,
    Kraus, A. and James, G.:
    The Anti-Coronary Club: A dietary approach to the prevention
    of coronary heart disease - a seven year report.
    Amer. J. Publ. Hlth. 56: 299, 1966.
33. Kagan, A., Dawber, T.R., Kannel, W.B. and Revotskie, N.:
    The Framingham study: a prospective study of coronary
    heart disease.
    Fed. Proc. 21, Suppl., 52, 1962.
34. Leren, P.:
    The effect of plasma cholesterol lowering diet in male
    survivors of myocardial infarction. Norwegian Monographs
    on Medical Science.
    Universitetsforlaget, Oslo, 1966.
35. The National Diet-Heart Study Final Report.
    Amer. Heart Ass. Monograph No. 18, 1968.
36. Dayton, S., Pearce, M.L., Hashimoto, S., Dixon, W.J.
    and Tomiyasu, U.:
    A controlled clinical trial of a diet high in unsaturated fat.
    Amer. Heart Ass. Monograph No. 25, 1969.
37. Turpeinen, O., Karvonen, M.J. and Roine, P.:
    Dietary prevention of coronary heart disease.
    Proc. 7th Int. Congr. Nutr., Hamburg, 1966, vol. 5, p. 361
    F. Vieweg & Sohn, Braunschweig, 1967.
38. Miettinen, M., Turpeinen, O., Karvonen, M.J., Elosuo, R.
    and Paavilainen, E.:
    Effect of cholesterol-lowering diet on mortality from
    coronary heart disease and other causes: A twelve-year
    clinical trial in men and women.
    Lancet, 2: 835, 1972.
39. Wolfram, G. und Zöllner, N.:
    Der Linolsäurebedarf des Menschen.
    Wiss. Veröffentl. der DGE, 22: 51, 1971.
40. Holman, R.T.:
    Essential fatty acid requirement.
    Fédération Int. Laiterie, An. Bull. II, 87, 1962.
41. Zöllner, N.:
    Personal communication.
42. Schettler, G., Kirsch, K., Kuhn, E., Knedel, M., Ott, H.,
    Schlüssel, H., Schölmerich, P. und Günther, W.:
    Die Vitamine A+E+B_6 in der Behandlung der Arteriosklerose.
    Dtsch. Med. Wschr., 85: 17, 734, 1960.
43. Shute, W.E. and Taub, H.J.:
    Vitamin E for ailing and healthy hearts.
    N.Y. Pyramid Books, 1972.
44. Weber, F., Weiser, H. und Wiss, O.:
    Bedarf an Vitamin E in Abhängigkeit von der Zufuhr
    an Linolsäure.
    Z. Ernährungsw. 4: 245, 1964.

45. Weber, F. und Weiser, H.:
    Vitamin E-Bedarf.
    Wiss. Veröff. Dtsch. Ges. Ernährung, 16: 137, 1967.
46. Schroeder, H.A.:
    Relation between mortality from cardiovascular disease
    and treated water supplies: variations in states in
    163 largest municipalities of the United States.
    J. Amer. Med. Ass. 172: 1902, 1960.
47. Morris, J.N., Crawford, M.D. and Heady, J.A.:
    Hardness of local water-supplies and mortality from
    cardiovascular disease in the county boroughs of
    England and Wales.
    Lancet, 1: 860, 1961.
48. Biörck, G., Bostrom, H. and Wistrom, A.:
    On the relationship between water hardness and death rate
    in cardiovascular diseases.
    Acta Med. Scand., 178: 239, 1965.
49. Masironi, R.:
    Cardiovascular mortality in relation to radioactivity and
    Hardness of local water supplies.
    Bull. WHO, 43: 687, 1970.
50. Kobayashi, J.:
    Geographical relationship between chemical nature of river
    water and death-rate from apoplexy.
    Ber. ohara Inst. Landw. Biol., 2: 12, 1957.
51. Masironi, R., Miesch, A.T., Crawford, M.D. and Hamilton, E.I.:
    Geochemical environments, trace elements, and cardiovascular
    diseases.
    Bull. WHO, 47: 139, 1972.
52. Bierenbaum, N.L., Fleischman, A.I., Dunn, J.P., Belk H.D.
    and Storter, B.M.:
    Serum lipids in hard and soft water communities.
    Israel J. Med. Sci., 5: 657, 1969.
53. Kamiyama, S., Yamada, F., Kobayashi, S. and Takahashi, E.:
    Comparative study on physical condition and blood chemistry
    of inhabitants in farm and fishing villages in relation to
    their difference in mortality from cerebrovascular disease.
    Tohoku, J. Exp. Med., 97: 81, 1969.
54. Seeling, M.S.:
    Myocardiology, p. 615 and 626 (edited by
    E. Bajusz and G. Rona, Baltimore, 1972).
55. Crawford, M.D.:
    Cardiovascular disease and water hardness:
    a review and assessment of evidence and possible
    mechanisms. WHO Meeting of investigators on trace
    elements in relation to cardiovascular diseases
    Joint WHO/IAEA research project, Geneva, 1973.

56. Stitt, F.W., Crawford, M.D., Clayton, D.G. and Morris, J.N.:
    Clinical and biochemical indicators of cardiovascular disease
    among men living in hard and soft water areas.
    Lancet, I, 122, 1973.
57. Schroeder, H.A. and Vinton, W.H. Jr.:
    Hypertension induced in rats by small doses of cadmium.
    Amer. J. Physiol., 202, 518, 1962.
58. Schroeder, H.A.:
    Cadmium as a factor in hypertension.
    J. Chron. Dis., 18: 647, 1965.
59. Schroeder, H.A., Nason, A.P. and Balassa, J.J.:
    Trace metals in rat tissues as influenced by calcium in water.
    J. Nutr., 93: 331, 1967.
60. Schroeder, H.A.:
    The role of chromium in mammalian nutrition.
    Amer. J. Clin. Nutr., 21: 230, 1968.
61. Kanabrocki, E.L., Case, L.F., Fields, T., Graham, L.,
    Miller, E.B., Oester, Y.T. and Kaplan, E.:
    Manganese and copper levels in human urine.
    J. Nucl. Med., 6: 780, 1965.
62. Kanabrocki, E.L., Case, L.F., Graham, L., Fields, T.,
    Miller, E.B., Oester, Y.T. and Kaplan, E.:
    Non-dialyzable manganese and copper levels in serum of patients
    with various diseases.
    J. Nucl. Med., 8: 166, 1967.
63. Harman, D.: Atherosclerosis: possible role of serum copper in
    the conversion of fatty streaks to fibrous plaques.
    Circulation, 34: Suppl. III, 13, 1966.
64. Harman, D.: Atherogenesis in minipigs: effect of dietary fat
    unsaturation and of copper.
    Circulation, 38: Suppl. VI, 8, 1968.
65. Coulson, W.F.:
    Kupfer und Arterien.
    CIBA Revue, p. 3, July 1973.
66. Mountain, J.T., Stockell, F.R. and Stokinger, H.E.:
    Effect of ingested vanadium on cholesterol and
    phospholipid metabolism in the rabbit.
    Proc. Soc. Exp. Biol. (N.Y.), 92: 582, 1956.
67. Schütte, K.:
    The biology of trace elements, London,
    Crosby Lockwood, p. 123, 1964.
68. Korkhov, V.V.:
    Vanadium in prophylaxis and treatment of experimental
    atherosclerosis.
    Farmakol. i Toksikol., 28: 83, 1965.
69. Schroeder, H.A., Vinton, W.H. Jr. and Balassa, J.J.:
    Effect of chromium, cadmium and other trace metals
    on the growth and survival of mice.
    J. Nutr., 80: 39, 1963.

70. Speckmann, E.W. and Brink, M.F.:
    Relationships between fat and mineral metabolism - A review.
    J. Amer. Diet. Ass., 51: 517, 1967.
71. Curran, G.L., Azarnoff, D.L. and Bolinger, R.E.:
    Effect of cholesterol synthesis inhibition in
    normocholesteremic young men.
    J. Clin. Invest., 38: 1251, 1959.
72. Schroeder, H.A.:
    Municipal drinking water and cardiovascular death rates.
    J. Amer. Med. Ass., 195: 81, 1966.
73. Fidanza, F.:
    Epidemiological evidence for the fat theory.
    Proc. Nutr. Soc., 31: 317, 1972.

THE EFFECTS OF FEEDING VARIOUS CARBOHYDRATES ON THE DEVELOPMENT OF HYPERCHOLESTEROLEMIA AND ATHEROSCLEROSIS

David Kritchevsky

The Wistar Institute of Anatomy and Biology

36th Street at Spruce, Philadelphia, Pa.   19104

Dietary carbohydrates affect serum lipid levels in man as well as in other species. In general, the ingestion of simple sugars is correlated with hyperlipemia, a phenomenon that has been the subject of several exhaustive reviews (1-4). The ingestion of sucrose has been linked to the development of heart disease in man (5-7).

Alfin-Slater (8) found that rats fed sucrose plus butter exhibited higher plasma cholesterol levels than did rats fed butter and either glucose or starch. When corn oil was the dietary fat, plasma cholesterol levels of the sucrose and starch groups were similar. Addition of cholesterol to the diet resulted in similar cholesterol levels (125-135 mg/dl) in rats fed butter and sucrose, glucose or starch. When corn oil was substituted for butter all cholesterol levels were lower (75-105 mg/dl) with greatest cholesterolemia observed in the glucose group. Staub and Thiessen (9) fed carbohydrates plus cholesterol to rats and found sucrose and fructose to be more cholesteremic than glucose or starch. However, Anderson (10) has reported that various types of raw starch are all more cholesteremic than sucrose. Grant and Fahrenbach (11) have found that sucrose is more cholesteremic than glucose in cholesterol fed chicks and rabbits. Pollak (12) found starch to be more cholesteremic than sucrose.

In experiments involving the establishment of atherosclerosis in animals fed cholesterol plus carbohydrates, Wells and Anderson (13) reported that lactose was significantly more atherogenic than sucrose in rabbits fed cholesterol.

O'Brien et al. (14) found starch and sucrose to be equally atherogenic in rabbits. A similar observation has been made in swine (15). Working with monkeys, Lang and Barthel (16) have shown that the cholesteremic and atherogenic response to dietary carbohydrate is different in different strains of monkey.

In 1958 and 1959, Lambert et al. (17) and Malmros and Wigand (18-20) reported that a semi-synthetic diet high in carbohydrate and saturated fat was atherogenic for rabbits. We had shown previously (21) that long term feeding of a chow-saturated fat diet was without atherogenic effect. Collation of the data (22) available in 1963 showed that cream (23), vegetable shortening (24), hydrogenated cottonseed oil (25) or coconut oil (26) were not atherogenic when added to a chow diet, even over long periods of feeding.

Saturated fat added to a semi-synthetic diet, on the other hand, led to atherosclerosis in rabbits (27-32). The atherogenic diets contained 21-55% carbohydrate, generally glucose or glucose plus sucrose. We set about to determine the role of specific carbohydrates in the semi-synthetic, atherogenic diet.

In our first experiment (33), we investigated the role of the fat present in chow. The standard diet contained 25 parts of Casein, 40 of dextrose, 5 of salt mix, 15 of cellulose, 1 of vitamin mix and 14 of hydrogenated coconut oil. Rabbit chow was extracted with ether-alcohol (1:1) and both the extract and residue were used. The diets and their designations are given in Table 1. The results (Table 2) show that the chow lipid did not affect cholesteremia or atherosclerosis and reaffirmed earlier findings that addition of coconut oil to chow does not affect atherosclerosis.

Having shown that the effect of the semi-synthetic diet was not easily altered, we began to compare the effects of different types of carbohydrate on cholesteremia and atherosclerosis in rabbits (34). In this experiment the carbohydrates fed were: glucose (G), sucrose (S), starch (T) and partially hydrolyzed starch (H). The results are presented in Table 3. It is evident the starch is the most atherogenic carbohydrate and glucose is the least.

In view of the reported atherogenicity of lactose in a cholesterol containing diet (13), we carried out another experiment testing this carbohydrate in a semi-synthetic diet (35). After four months of feeding of the diet (Table 4), it was seen that sucrose, fructose and starch were more atherogenic than either glucose or lactose. At ten months (Table 5) the order of athero-

TABLE 1

Composition of Diets Fed to Rabbits

Ingredient	Diet designation					
	SS	SS-PF	XP-HCNO	SS-LA	PC-HCNO	PC
Casein	25	25	--	25	--	--
Dextrose	40	40	--	40	--	--
Salt mix[a]	5	5	--	5	--	--
Cellulose	15	15	--	15	--	--
Vitamin mix[b]	1	1	1	1	--	--
Hydrogenated coconut oil	14	12	14	13	12	--
Lauric acid	--	--	--	1	--	--
Purina chow fat	--	2	--	--	--	--
Purina chow residue	--	--	85	--	--	--
Purina chow	--	--	--	--	88	100

[a]Salt mix, USP XIV, (percent): $Al_2 (SO_4)_3 \cdot (NH_4)_2SO_4 \cdot 24H_2O$ (0.009); $CaHPO_4 \cdot 2 H_2O$ (11.28); $CaCO_3$ (6.86), $Ca_3 (C_6H_5O_7)_2 \cdot 4 H_2O$ (30.83); $CuSO_4$ (0.008); $Fe(NH_4) (C_6H_5O_7)_2$ (1.526); $MgCO_3$ (3.520); $MgSO_4$ (3.83); $MnSO_4$ (0.02); KCl (12.47); KI (0.004); KH_2PO_4 (21.88); NaCl (7.71); NaF (0.05).

[b]Vitamin Mix (g/kg diet): p-aminobenzoic acid (0.11); vitamin C (1.017); biotin (0.0004); Ca pantothenate (0.066); choline citrate (3.715); folic acid (0.002); inositol (0.11); vitamin K (0.05); nicotinic acid (0.009); pyridoxine $\cdot$ HCl (0.022); riboflavin (0.022); thiamine $\cdot$ HCl (0.002); vitamin A, 500,000 U/g (0.039); vitamin B_{12} (0.029); vitamin D_2, 500,000 U/g (0.004); vitamin E acetate, 250 U/g (0.485).

TABLE 2

Influence of Special Diets on Cholesteremia and
Atherosclerosis in Rabbits

Diet	Cholesterol		L/B	Atherosclerosis	
	Serum (mg/dl)	Liver (mg/100g)	Lipoprotein Cholesterol	Arch	Thoracic
SS	207±36	1111±137	0.15	1.2	0.5
SS-PF	249±41	829±77	0.24	1.1	0.7
XP-HCNO	64±9	599±37	0.24	0.5	0.3
SS-LA	207±36	931±74	0.17	1.4	0.6
PC-HCNO	35±2	466±24	0.37	0.3	0.2
PC	40±9	318±22	0.39	0.2	0.1

TABLE 3

Influence of Dietary Carbohydrates on Cholesteremia
and Atherosclerosis in Rabbits

Diet	Cholesterol		L/B	Atherosclerosis	
	Serum (mg/dl)	Liver (mg/100g)	Lipoprotein Cholesterol	Arch	Thoracic
G	209±31	1.66±0.03	0.17	1.1	0.9
S	310±66	1.23±0.18	0.05	1.9	1.0
T	640±97	1.90±0.27	0.03	2.3	1.2
H	400±77	1.31±0.24	0.05	1.7	1.0
Control	57±10	0.33±0.03	0.39	0.0	0.0

TABLE 4

Influence of Semi-Synthetic Diets on Rabbits
(4 Months)

| GP | Cholesterol | | Triglycerides | | Atheromata | |
	Serum (mg/dl)	Liver (g/100g)	Serum	Liver	Arch	Thoracic
Glucose	193	0.69	134	1.26	0.6	0.4
Fructose	177	0.83	190	1.38	0.9	0.8
Sucrose	181	0.70	105	1.07	1.0	0.7
Lactose	155	0.83	107	1.67	0.6	0.3
Starch	138	0.71	114	1.16	0.8	0.5
Control	46	0.27	98	0.94	0.0	0.0

TABLE 5

Influence of Semi-Synthetic Diets on Rabbits
(10 Months)

| GP | Cholesterol | | Triglycerides | | Atheromata | |
	Serum (mg/dl)	Liver (g/100g)	Serum	Liver	Arch	Thoracic
Glucose	451	1.62	92	0.22	1.1	0.6
Fructose	922	1.91	116	0.26	2.1	0.9
Sucrose	520	1.69	248	0.21	1.7	1.2
Lactose	329	1.81	107	0.71	0.6	0.4
Starch	532	2.01	254	0.41	1.5	1.2

genicity of the dietary carbohydrates was fructose, sucrose, starch, glucose, lactose.

We then turned our attention to the possible atherogenic effects of this diet in other species. We chose to study this diet in baboons, a species which can be rendered atherogenic on a cholesterol-containing regimen (36).

Five groups of six baboons each (three male, three female) were used. The baboons were fed semi-synthetic diets containing glucose, fructose, sucrose and starch. A control group was maintained on the laboratory regimen of bread, bananas, yams, oranges and carrots. The animals were fed for one year at which time they were killed, the aortas graded for sudanophilia and the lipid content of various organs determined. Two baboons from each group were used to measure cholesterol synthesis from labeled mevalonic acid before and after the feeding experiment. Full details of the analytical and histological methodologies are published elsewhere (37).

It is evident from Table 6 that the semi-synthetic regimen was hypercholesteremic as well as hypertriglyceredemic. The average increase in triglyceride levels was higher in the groups fed fructose and sucrose (49-65%) than it was in the groups fed starch and glucose (35-38%). The fatty acid spectrum of the serum lipids (Table 7) reflected the nature of the dietary fat. The liver lipids of the baboons on the test diets showed increased levels of triglycerides and ester cholesterol (Table 8). These changes would be expected upon feeding of a hyperlipemic regimen. The liver fatty acids (Table 9), like the serum fatty acids, reflected the influence of dietary coconut oil. The control liver lipids contained less lauric and myristic acids than did the liver lipids of the test groups.

All of the test diets led to aortic sudanophilia (Table 10). The average sudanophilia was highest in the group fed fructose and lowest in that fed glucose. If the severity of sudanophilia is ranked by the method of Wilcoxon (38), the average rankings were: fructose--66.5; sucrose--64.5; starch--87.0; glucose--86.0; and control--161.0. The females fed fructose and sucrose exhibited more severe sudanophilia than did the males, and the reverse was true in the groups fed starch and glucose. The aortic lipids (Table 11) are similar in all five groups, possibly reflecting the fact that only fatty streaking was observed. The free/ester cholesterol levels of atherosclerotic aortas are generally much lower than those of normal aortas (39).

Table 12 summarizes the serum and liver lipids of baboons in each group with greatest or least sudanophilia. It is evident

TABLE 6

Average Serum Lipid Values of Baboons Fed Special Diets
For 12 Months

Diet	Cholesterol (mg/dl) (121)*	Triglycerides (mg/dl) (75)	β-Lipoprotein Cholesterol (%) (55)
Fructose	162±10**a	129±11a	66±1.1a
Sucrose	152± 9a	116± 8a	65±1.3a
Starch	156± 8a	108± 5a	64±1.0a
Glucose	151±11b	105± 7a	63±1.0a
Control	113± 3	78± 4	57±1.0

* Average starting levels, all animals.
** Standard Error
   Significance, diet vs control: a p < 0.001; b p < 0.01.

TABLE 7

Average Fatty Acids of Baboon Serum Lipids

Group	Fatty Acid						
	12:0	14:0	16:0	16:1	18:0	18:1	18:2
Fructose							
CEFA*	-	1.6	28.3	10.8	14.3	36.3	8.5
TGFA**	1.7	4.4	44.4	5.0	8.7	36.1	tr
TFA***	tr	3.2	36.4	4.5	15.1	30.9	9.1
Sucrose							
CEFA	-	2.0	31.5	10.8	14.3	33.9	7.7
TGFA	tr	3.9	45.1	4.1	8.6	37.6	tr
TFA	tr	3.1	40.3	4.9	14.1	31.1	6.6
Starch							
CEFA	-	2.6	32.8	10.6	13.4	29.8	11.0
TGFA	tr	3.7	49.0	4.6	9.2	33.2	tr
TFA	tr	2.3	39.6	4.6	15.5	25.4	12.8
Glucose							
CEFA	-	3.2	35.7	10.6	16.7	29.0	5.2
TGFA	2.0	4.8	44.2	4.8	12.0	32.4	tr
TFA	tr	3.2	35.7	5.4	17.2	28.0	10.0
Control							
CEFA	-	0.8	27.0	2.3	12.8	32.7	24.4
TGFA	-	tr	45.9	1.5	8.9	34.5	9.8
TFA	-	tr	38.1	tr	17.5	24.0	20.5

  * Cholesteryl ester fatty acids
 ** Triglyceride fatty acids
*** Total fatty acids

TABLE 8

Liver Lipids of Baboons (mg/gm ± SEM)

	FC	EC	FC/EC	TG	PL
Fructose	1.97±.28	2.79±.44	0.71	3.69± .68	23.15±1.61
Sucrose	1.76±.18	2.86±.43	0.62	5.93±1.82	24.85± .49
Starch	2.17±.20	3.21±.79	0.68	9.58±2.19	24.58± .79
Glucose	1.92±.19	2.89±.43	0.66	8.66±2.96	21.95±1.28
Control	1.78±.15	1.66±.28	1.07	3.46±1.05	22.38±1.40

FC - free cholesterol   TG - triglycerides
EC - esterified cholesterol   PL - phospholipids

TABLE 9

Fatty Acid Content of Baboon Livers

| Diet Group | Fraction | \multicolumn{8}{c}{Fatty Acid} |
		12:0	14:0	16:0	16:1	18:0	18:1	18:2	18:3
Fructose	CEFA*	-	2.6	34.7	5.8	22.5	26.1	2.6	3.2
	TGFA**	3.9	7.7	51.3	2.8	12.5	19.0	1.6	1.3
	TFA***	1.8	4.8	31.1	8.1	18.9	29.2	6.0	-
Sucrose	CEFA	-	4.1	37.0	9.8	19.6	21.1	3.0	1.7
	TGFA	2.2	6.2	59.4	3.0	9.2	19.1	1.5	0.9
	TFA	4.5	4.8	32.5	8.4	16.6	28.6	7.8	-
Starch	CEFA	-	3.8	37.3	12.1	16.3	26.8	3.5	0.7
	TGFA	4.6	10.0	49.9	4.1	10.1	21.5	tr	-
	TFA	2.6	6.3	32.1	8.2	14.2	28.6	9.2	-
Glucose	CEFA	-	4.5	36.1	11.5	16.3	27.4	3.7	0.7
	TGFA	4.0	9.0	44.5	6.2	8.1	28.5	tr	-
	TFA	3.3	8.1	31.3	10.6	13.1	30.5	3.4	-
Control	CEFA	-	-	28.6	2.8	20.3	36.9	8.9	2.0
	TGFA	-	0.7	40.6	2.6	12.7	36.2	7.4	-
	TFA	-	tr	29.9	3.3	16.8	28.9	21.4	-

*Cholesteryl ester fatty acids
**Triglyceride fatty acids
***Total fatty acids

TABLE 10

Percent of Aorta Area Stained With Sudan IV

Sex	Fructose	Sucrose	Starch	Glucose	Control
F	35.0	30.0	15.0	1.0	0.0
F	10.0	2.0	0.1	0.5	0.0
F	0.5	1.0	0.0	0.2	0.0
M	20.0	3.0	25.0	30.0	0.1
M	1.0	3.0	15.0	5.0	0.0
M	0.5	1.0	0.5	0.5	0.0
Avg. ±SEM	11.2±5.7	6.7±4.7	9.3±4.3	6.2±4.8	0.02±0.02

TABLE 11

Aorta Lipids of Baboons (mg/gm ± SEM)

	FC	EC	FC/EC	TG	PL
Fructose	0.61±.06	0.34±.07	1.79	1.32±.20	5.89±.17
Sucrose	0.59±.05	0.20±.03	2.95	1.28±.39	6.03±.54
Starch	0.78±.07	0.41±.11	1.90	1.31±.29	6.53±.42
Glucose	0.53±.06	0.34±.06	1.56	0.96±.25	4.71±.62
Control	0.73±.06	0.39±.16	1.87	1.10±.21	5.30±.49

TABLE 12

Serum and Liver Lipid Levels in Baboons in Each Group
With Greatest or Least Aortic Sudanophilia

GP.	Sex	Sudanophilia (%)	Serum (mg/dl)		Liver (mg/gm)	
			Cholesterol	Triglyceride	Cholesterol	Triglyceride
F	F	35.0	153	130	5.43	3.86
F	F	0.5	128	89	3.29	1.46
SU	F	30.0	133	255	4.64	4.76
SU	M	1.0	142	134	7.12	12.62
ST	M	25.0	102	115	4.42	14.24
ST	F	0.0	107	296	4.34	6.94
G	M	30.0	165	123	3.23	0.48
G	F	0.2	157	147	6.61	13.76
C	M	0.1	97	153	3.40	4.20
C	F	0.0	110	131	8.85	7.64

that, in this very limited sample, no correlations are seen between sudanophilia and lipemia.

The characteristics of the two cholesterol biosynthesis experiments are shown in Table 13. The major differences were the slower appearance of ester cholesterol in the baboons fed fructose and sucrose. These differences might be due to the different isotopes used or to the fact that the animals had aged one year. Since these data are derived from only two animals it is difficult to draw conclusions, but the effect of dietary fructose and sucrose upon rates of cholesterol esterification merits further study.

The biliary bile acids were primarily present as the taurine conjugates. The complete bile acid spectra of the pooled biles are presented in Table 14. Analysis of biliary lipid radioactivity indicates that the ratio of cholesterol to cholanoic acid specific activity is much higher in the test groups than in the controls (Table 15). These data suggest reduced conversion of cholesterol to bile acids. The ratio of primary (cholic and chenodeoxycholic) to secondary (lithocholic and deoxycholic) bile acids was highest in the control group, also suggesting reduced synthesis of bile acids (Table 16). One source of the hypercholesteremia observed in animals fed semi-synthetic diets may be a reduced conversion of cholesterol to bile acids, with the "excess" sterol thus available entering the circulation. Kyd and Bouchier (40) recently reached a similar conclusion based on data obtained in rabbits fed a lithogenic diet.

In summary, semi-synthetic diets containing saturated fat are more cholesteremic, β-lipoproteinemic and atherogenic than "natural" diets. When different carbohydrates are used in semi-synthetic diets fructose and sucrose are more atherogenic than glucose. This effect has been observed in rabbits and baboons. Semi-synthetic diets appear to exert an inhibitory effect on bile acid synthesis and this may explain partially the hypercholesteremic properties of these diets.

TABLE 13

Summary of Characteristics of Cholesterol Biosynthesis Curves

Dietary Group	Curve Characteristic	Expt. 1** (HRS)	Expt. 2** (HRS)	Change (HRS)
Fructose	Peak Free SA*	6.5	9.0	+ 2.5
	Crossover	31.6	34.0	+ 2.4
	Peak Ester SA	43	48	+ 5.0
Sucrose	Peak Free SA	5.3	10.0	+ 4.7
	Crossover	40.4	59.2	+ 18.8
	Peak Ester SA	45	56	+ 11.0
Starch	Peak Free SA	5.3	8.0	+ 2.7
	Crossover	38.2	33.1	- 5.1
	Peak Ester SA	41	34	- 7.0
Glucose	Peak Free SA	5.0	9.0	+ 4.0
	Crossover	32.5	33.4	+ 0.9
	Peak Ester SA	36	35	- 1.0
Control	Peak Free SA	5.0	7.3	+ 2.3
	Crossover	22.7	20.2	- 2.5
	Peak Ester SA	31	27	- 4.0

 * SA - specific activity, dpm/mg
** Experiments carried out one year apart
   Precursors: Expt. 1 - [2-^{14}C] mevalonic acid
                Expt. 2 - [5-^{3}H] mevalonic acid

TABLE 14

Biliary Bile Acid Spectrum* (mg/ml)

Diet	Taurine Conjugates					Glycine Conjugates				
	Total	L	D	CD	C	Total	L	D	CD	C
Fructose	31.3	0.9	19.1	6.2	5.1	0.53	.03	.34	.10	.06
Sucrose	28.9	1.0	16.2	7.0	4.7	3.02	.23	2.29	.47	.03
Starch	48.8	1.3	19.4	12.8	15.3	1.11	.05	.63	.34	.09
Glucose	39.4	1.3	20.2	10.1	7.8	1.83	.02	1.23	.47	.11
Control	39.3	1.1	13.4	8.5	16.3	1.35	.11	.61	.45	.18

L - Lithocholic Acid
D - Deoxycholic Acid
CD - Chenodeoxycholic Acid
C - Cholic Acid

TABLE 15

Specific Activity (dpm/mg x 10^3) of Bile Lipids of Baboons
Given [5-^{3}H] Mevalonate

Product	Dietary Group				
	Fructose	Sucrose	Starch	Glucose	Control
Cholesterol	88	30	47	47	59
Taurocholanoic Acids	3	3	2	2	15
Glycocholanoic Acids	5	3	3	5	15

TABLE 16

Ratio of Primary/Secondary Bile Acids (P/S)

Dietary Groups	P/S Ratios		
	Taurine Conjugates	Glycine Conjugates	Total Bile Acids
Fructose	0.57	0.43	0.56
Sucrose	0.68	0.20	0.61
Starch	1.36	0.63	1.33
Glucose	0.83	0.46	0.81
Control	1.71	0.88	1.67

Primary bile acids - cholic and chenodeoxycholic
Secondary bile acids - lithocholic and deoxycholic

SUMMARY

It is possible to establish atherosclerosis in rabbits by feeding semi-synthetic diets that are high in carbohydrate and saturated fat and devoid of cholesterol. Addition of saturated fat to laboratory chow does not render the chow atherogenic. When rabbits were fed diets which differ only in the carbohydrate component, starch was found to be more atherogenic than sucrose which, in turn, was more atherogenic than glucose. All the diets were hypercholesteremic and hypertriglyceridemic. In another series of experiments diets containing fructose or sucrose were more atherogenic than diets containing glucose, lactose or sorbitol.

Baboons were fed semi-synthetic diets containing fructose, sucrose, starch or glucose (but no cholesterol) for one year. Serum cholesterol levels were 155-165 mg/dl in all test groups. The normal baboon cholesterol level is 115 mg/dl. Serum trigly-cerides were elevated from the normal level of 73 mg/dl to about 110 mg/dl in the groups fed starch and glucose and to about 125 mg/dl in the groups fed fructose and sucrose. Liver and lung cholesterol ester levels were also raised. The test groups all showed aortic sudanophilia. The most severe sudanophilia was observed in the fructose group (11.2% of surface area) and the least in the glucose group (6.2% of surface area).

The biliary cholesterol specific activities (after administration of [^{3}H]-mevalonic acid) were the same in all groups, but biliary bile acid specific activity was higher in the control baboons than in test animals. These data, plus the higher primary/secondary bile acid ratio observed in the test animals, suggest that reduced bile acid synthesis may be one cause of the hyper-cholesteremia observed in animals fed the semi-synthetic diets.

ACKNOWLEDGMENTS

This work was supported, in part, by Public Health Service Research Grants HL03299 and HL05209 and Research Career Award 0734 from the National Heart and Lung Institute; RR05540 from the Division of Research Resources, and Research Grant 82 from the National Dairy Council.

REFERENCES

1. Hodges, R.E. and Krehl, W.A.
    Am. J. Clin. Nutr. 17: 334, 1965.
2. Macdonald, I.
    Advances in Lipid Research,
    Vol. 4 (ed. R. Paoletti and D. Kritchevsky)
    Academic Press, N.Y. 1966, p. 39.
3. McGandy, R.B., Hegsted, D.M. and Stare, F.J.
    New England J. Med. 227: 417, 1967.
4. Macdonald, I.
    World Rev. Nutr. Diet 8: 143, 1967.
5. Yudkin, J.
    Proc. Nutr. Soc. 23: 149, 1964.
6. Yudkin, J. and Morland, J.
    Am. J. Clin. Nutr. 20: 503, 1967.
7. Yudkin, J.
    Proc. Nutr. Soc. 31: 331, 1972.
8. Alfin-Slater, R.B.
    J. Dairy Sci. 50: 781, 1967.
9. Staub, H.W. and Thiessen, R. Jr.
    J. Nutrition 95: 633, 1968.
10. Anderson T.A.
    Proc. Soc. Exp. Biol. Med. 130: 884, 1969.
11. Grant, W.C. and Fahrenbach, J.
    Proc. Soc. Exp. Biol. Med. 100: 250, 1959.
12. Pollak, O.J.
    J. Am. Geriatrics Soc. 9: 349, 1961.
13. Wells, W.W. and Anderson, S.C.
    J. Nutrition 68: 541, 1959.
14. O'Brien, S., Pond, W.G. and Krook, L.
    Nutrition Reports Int. 5: 213, 1972.
15. St. Clair, R.W., Bullock, B.C. Lehner, N.D.M.,
    Clarkson, T.B. and Lofland H.B. Jr.
    Exper. Molec. Pathol. 15: 21, 1971.
16. Lang, C.M. and Barthel, C.H.
    Am. J. Clin. Nutr. 25: 470, 1972.
17. Lambert, G.F., Miller, J.P., Olsen, R.T. and Frost, D.V.
    Proc. Soc. Exp. Biol. Med. 97: 544, 1958.
18. Malmros, H. and Wigand, G.
    Lancet ii: 749, 1959.
19. Wigand, G.
    Acta Med. Scand. 166: Suppl. 351, 1959.
20. Malmros, H. and Wigand, G.
    Z. Ernahrungwiss 1: 20, 1960.
21. Kritchevsky, D. and Tepper, S.A.
    J. Atheroscler. Res. 4: 113, 1964.
22. Kritchevsky, D.
    J. Atheroscler. Res. 4: 103, 1964.

23. Hirsch, E.F. and Nailor, R.
    Arch. Pathol. 59: 419, 1955.
24. Kritchevsky, D. Moyer, A.W., Tesar, W.C., Logan, J.B.
    Brown, R.A., Davies, M.C. and Cox, H.R.
    Am. J. Physiol. 178: 30, 1954.
25. Van Handel, E. and Zilversmit, D.B.
    Circulation 16: 516, 1957.
26. Steiner, A., Varsos, A. and Samuel, P.
    Circulation Res. 7: 448, 1959.
27. Gottenbos, J.J. and Thomasson, H.J.
    Colloq. Int. Centre Nat. Rech. Sci. (Paris) 99: 221, 1961
28. Funch, J.P., Krogh, B. and Dam, H.
    Brit. J. Nutr. 14: 355, 1960.
29. Brechter, C.L. and Forsby, N.H.
    Z. Ernahrungswiss 3: 95, 1962.
30. Funch, J.P., Kristensen, G. and Dam, H.
    Brit. J. Nutr. 16: 497, 1962.
31. Gresham, G.A. and Howard, A.N.
    Arch. Pathol. 74: 1, 1962.
32. Moore, J.H. and Kon, S.K.
    Chem. Ind. (London) p. 165, 1963.
33. Kritchevsky, D. and Tepper, S.A.
    J. Atheroscler. Res. 8: 357, 1968.
34. Kritchevsky, D., Sallata, P. and Repper, S.A.
    J. Atheroscler. Res. 8: 697, 1968.
35. Kritchevsky, D., Tepper, S.A. and Kitagawa, M.
    Nutr. Reports Int. 7: 193, 1973.
36. Strong, J.P. and McGill, H.C. Jr.
    Am. J. Pathol. 50: 669, 1967.
37. Kritchevsky, D., Davidson, L.M., Shapiro, I.L., Kim, H.K.,
    Kitagawa, M., Malhotra, S., Nair, P.P., Clarkson, T.B.,
    Bersohn, I. and Winter, P.A.D.
    Am. J. Clin. Nutr.,
    In press
38. Wilcoxon, F.
    Biometrics Bull. 1: 80, 1945.
39. Kritchevsky, D.
    Atherosclerotic Vascular Disease
    (ed. A. N. Brest and J.H. Moyer), Appleton-Century-Crofts,
    New York, p. 1, 1967.
40. Kyd, P.A. and Bouchier, I.A.D.
    Proc. Soc. Exp. Biol. Med. 141: 846, 1972.

INDEX

Acetyl CoA carboxylase, 6-9
Acetylsalicylic acid, 82
Actomyosin, 95, 99, 101
Acyl CoA synthetase, 8
Adenosine diphosphate (ADP),
    82, 110, 197
Adenosine monophosphate,
    cyclic (cAMP), 101
Adenosine monophosphate
    phosphodiesterase,
    101
  inhibitors, 77-105
Adenosine triphosphate (ATP)
    citrate lyase, 7, 9
Adrenal gland, weight of,
    47, 52
Albumin, 112
Alcohol, see Ethanol
Angiography, 122
Angiopathy, diabetic, 94
Angiotensin II, 79, 92, 96
Anti-Coronary Club Study,
    213
Aorta
  in cockerel, 40, 41
  intima, 87-88
  in monkey, 20-28
  thoracic, 91
Arachidonic acid, 68, 197
Artery
  carotid, 90
  coronary, 42-45, 48
Atheroma
  assessment, 119-120,
    122-123
  ruptured, 113

Atherosclerosis
  and age, 20
  and alcohol, 176-177
  angiography, 120
  animal model, lack of, 11
    monkey, 14-30
  aortic, 38
  caloric intake, 173, 175
  and carbohydrate intake, 13,
    57-64, 175-176, 231-250
  and cardiovascular complication,
    13
  and cockerels, 33
  coronary, 38
  development, 65-77
  diagnostic methods, 119-124
    angiography, 120
    flow dependent, 120
    ischemia detection, 120-122
    roentgenography, 120
  and diet, 13-31
    American, 69-72
  etiology, 151-514, 172
  and exercise, 33-56
  fat, dietary, types of, 173-175
    intake, 65-77
  fructose, 59, 206
  and Macaca nigra, 14-30
  and minerals, 177-178
  and monkey, 14-30, 65
  and nutrition, 125
  and obesity, 125, 206
  and overweight, see Obesity
  prevention by diet, 171-189,
    205-230
  and protein level, 177

Atherosclerosis (cont'd)
  regression, 65-77
  risk factors, 78, 125-158,
      206
    cigarette smoking, see
        Smoking
    hypercholesterolemia, 78
    hypertension, see
        Hypertension
  sucrose, 206
  swine model, 65
  theory of contraction of
      endothelial cells,
      77-105
  treatment with cAMP
      phosphodiesterase
      inhibitors, 77-105
  and vitamins, 178-179

Baboon
  aorta lipids, 241
  diet, 236-247
  fatty acid, 238, 240
  liver lipids, 239
Bacitracin, 10
Behenic acid, 68
Beta cell, loss of, 17-20, 30
Bile acid, 243, 244
Blood coagulation, 107-118
  pathway to, extrinsic,
      107-108
    intrinsic, 107-108
  schema, 108
Blood pressure, elevated,
      139-142
Bradykinin, 77, 92
Butter fat, 66, 67, 193, 231
Butter oil, 66

Cadmium, 177, 222, 223
Calcium, 222
Carbohydrate
  and atherosclerosis, 13,
      57-64, 175-176,
      231-250
  and cholesterol, 60, 61
  dietary, 57
    and triglyceride
        level, 58-59

Celebes black ape, 13
Celebes Island, location, 15
Cerulenin, 10
Chicago Heart Association
        Detection Project in
        Industry, 145-149
Cholesterol, 35, 37, 39, 51, 60,
        61, 77, 126-128, 131, 132,
        135-139, 144, 207, 208,
        234-237, 242-245
  and age, 211-212
  and atherosclerosis, 71
  biosynthesis, control of, 2
  in blood, 159, 163, 164
  and carbohydrate, 60, 61
  content of food, 210
  dietary, 159-163
  and egg intake, 209
  excretory routes, 160
  homeostasis, 161
  loading, 77, 94
  and obesity, 166-170
  in plasma, 33-34
  and sunflower oil, 214
  and Swedish men, 165
  turnover, daily, 168
Choline, 194
Chromium, 178, 223
Chylomicronemia, 139
Cigarette smoking, see Smoking
Citrate, 6, 7
Clofibrate, 5
Cockerel
  adrenal weight, 47, 52
  heart weight, 46
  Hy-line, 34
  thyroid weight, 47
Coconut oil, 66, 67, 68, 232, 236
Collagen, 49, 50, 73, 110, 197
  to elastin ratio, 33, 48, 53
  hydroxyproline, 33, 35, 48,
      50, 52
  nitrogen content, 35, 48, 50
Copper, 223
Corn oil, 66, 162, 164, 215, 231
Coronary Drug Project, 134
Cottonseed oil, 232
Cream, 232
Cytochrome P-450, 4

2,3-Decadienoyl-N-
        acetylcysteamine, 10
3-Decanoyl-N-
        acetylcysteamine, 10
7-Dehydro-cholesterol
        reductase, 4
Diabetes, juvenile, in
        Macaca nigra, 16, 20
Diet, see Atherosclerosis
Dolichol, 1, 2

Edematous arterial
        reaction, 79
EG 467, 82, 83, 98-100
Egg intake, 209
Elastin, 26, 35, 52, 53
  to collagen ratio, 33, 48,
        49, 53
Endothelial cell
  contractile protein, 92,
        94, 98
  contraction theory, 77,
        102
  pinch, 95
  of rabbit aorta, 84-86,
        89, 90
  and thrombus formation,
        98
Enzyme suicide, 10
Epinephrine, 77, 92
Equilenine, 2
Equilin, 2
Estradiol, 52
Ethanol, 176-177
  and fat, 167
  and triglyceride, 166
Ethanolamine, 194
Exercise
  and atherosclerosis,
        33-56
  and body weight, 35-36

Factor XI, 109
Farnesylpyrophosphate, 3
Fat, 60, 127
  and atherosclerosis, 65-77
  intake of saturated,
        128-131

Fatty acid, 109, 238
  dietary, 162
  platelet, 112
  polyunsaturated, 68, 173, 194,
        209, 213
  saturated, 173
Fatty acid synthetase, 8, 9
Fatty acyl CoA synthetase, 8
Feedback control, negative, 2
Ferritin, 95, 96
Fibrin, 99
Finnish Heart Study, 213, 215
Framingham Study, 134, 213
Fredrickson's type IV
        hyperlipoproteinemia, 59
Fructose, 59, 236, 238, 239,
        244-246

Glucose, 58, 238, 240, 244-246
Glucose-6-phosphate dehydrogenase,
        7
Glycerophospholipid, 200
Glycine, 246
Glycocholanic acid, 245
Glycolipid, 1

Heart disease, coronary
  risk factors, 207
  and sucrose, 231-232
Heart weight, 46
HMG-CoA, see β-Hydroxy-β-
        methylglutaryl CoA
Hydroxycitrate, 3
β-Hydroxy-β-methylglutaryl CoA   2
β-Hydroxy-β-methylglutaryl CoA
        reductase, 2, 3
Hydroxyproline, 33, 35, 48-52
Hyperbetalipoproteinemia, 138
Hypercholesterolemia, 65-78, 140,
        143, 144, 171
  and carbohydrate intake,
        231-250
Hypercoagulation
  and dietary fat, 191-204
Hyperemia, 121
Hyperglycemia, 125-158
Hypertriglyceridemia, 59, 170, 175
  ethanol, 177

Hyperinsulinemia, 20
Hyperlipidemia, 77, 111,
        112, 125-158
    and sugar intake, 231
Hyperlipoproteinemia, 79
    carbohydrate-induced, 59
    Fredrickson's type IV, 59
Hypertension, 78, 125-158,
        207

Immunoglobulin G, 96
Insulin, 7, 13, 16, 19, 30, 58
    immunoreactive, 17
    see Hyperinsulinemia
International Atherosclerosis
        Project, 126, 140
International Cooperative
        Study on the
        Epidemiology of
        Cardiovascular
        Disease, 126,
        129-132, 140
Ischemia, 120
    detection of, 120-122
Isocitric dehydrogenase, 7
Italian Society of
        Atherosclerosis
        Studies, 182

β-Ketoacyl thiolase, 3

Lactose, 231, 232
Langerhans, isle of, 18-22
Lathyrism, 94
Lauric acid, 174, 236
Linoleic acid, 193, 194,
        197
Lipid
    biosynthesis, control of,
        1-12
    and diet, 159-170
    of plasma, 159-170
Lipogenic system, 5
β-Lipoprotein, 77, 80, 96, 97
    low-density, 4

Macaca maura, 15
    M. nemestrina, 15
    M. nigra, 14-30

Magnesium, 222
Map, metabolic, 1
Margarine, 194
Metamorphosis, viscous, 108
Mortality
    and cholesterol, 127
    and fat, 127
Mycobacterium phlei synthetase, 9
Myristic acid, 174, 236

National Cooperative Pooling
        Project, 134, 135, 140,
        141, 143
National Diet Heart Study (in the
        U.S.A.), 213
Nephropathy, 94
Nicotinic acid, 178
Norepinephrine, 77

Obesity, 125, 166-170, 206
Oleic acid, 193
    synthesis, 8
Olive oil, 128, 215
Oxygenase, mixed function type, 4

Palmitaldehyde, 200
Palmitic acid, 174, 194
Palmitoyl CoA, 6, 9
Palmitoyl CoA thioesterase, 8
Pathway
    control of branched, 3
    multivariate repression, 3
    of sterol, 3
PDC, 100, 101
Peanut oil, 66, 68
Phagocytosis, 111
Phosphatidylethanolamine, 197-199
Phosphatidylinositol, 192
Phosphatidylserine, 192, 195
Phonoangiography, 121, 122
Phospholipase A_2, 200
Pinch phenomenon of endothelial
        cells, 95, 97
Plasmalogen, 200
Platelet
    activation, 107, 109-112
    aggregation, 99, 100
    composition, 201
    fatty acid metabolism, 112

Platelet (cont'd)
  and prostaglandin, 112
  and thrombosis, 107-118
Plethysmography, 121
Potassium, 177
Prebetalipoprotein, 17, 19,
        77, 80, 97
Premarin, 98
Prostaglandin, 1, 112
Protein factor, soluble, 4
Purina chow diet,
        composition of, 16
Pyridinolcarbamate, 79, 82,
        93

Rabbit diet, 233, 234
Rhesus monkey
  and atherosclerosis, 65
  and American diet, 69-72
Roentgenography, 122

Safflower oil, 194, 215
Serine phosphoglyceride, 194
Serotonin, 77, 92, 99
Shimamoto's theory of
        atherosclerosis,
        77-105
Smoking, cigarette, 137, 140,
        143, 144, 152, 207
Sodium chloride, 177
Soybean oil, 194, 215
SPF, see Protein factor,
        soluble
Sphingomyelin, 197
Squalene, 2, 4, 10
Squalene epoxidase, 4
Squalene epoxide, 4
Starch, 232, 236-241, 244-246
Stearaldehyde, 200
Stearic acid, 174, 193, 194
Sterol
  fecal excretion, 164
  pathway, control of, 3
Sterol carrier protein, 4
Sucrose, 128, 133, 206, 236,
        239-241, 244-246
  and heart disease, 231, 232
Sunflower oil, 196, 213-215,
        218-200
Swine model, 65

Taurine, 246
Taurocholanic acid, 245
Thioesterase, 9
Thiolase synthetase, 3
Thrombin, 110, 113, 197
Thromboplastin, 109
Thrombosis
  in animal, 191
  and blood coagulation, 107-118
  and fat, dietary, 191-204
  and fatty acid, 107-118
  and lipid, 107-118
  and platelet, 107-118
  by Salmonella typhi
        lipopolysaccharide, 192
Thrombus
  red, 113
  white, 113
Transacylation, 8
Triglyceride, 17, 19, 57-59, 139,
        235, 237, 242
  and alcohol, 166, 167
  and carbohydrate, dietary, 58-59
  and fructose, 59
  of plasma, 162-166
  and Swedish men, 165
Trojan horse effect, 10

Ubiquinone, 2

Vanadium, 223
Vegetable shortening, 232
Viscous metamorphosis, 108
Vitamin A, 178, 218, 221
  B_6, 178, 221
  C, 178
  E, 178, 219, 221
  niacin, 221
  pyridoxin, 218

Washing board phenomenon, 99, 100
Water hardness, 177, 221, 222
Wheat germ oil, 215

Yeast synthetase, 9

Zymosan, 110